THE EPIDEMIOLOGY OF COMMON HEALTH CONDITIONS AMONG ADULTS WITH DEVELOPMENTAL DISABILITIES IN PRIMARY CARE

THE EPIDEMIOLOGY OF COMMON HEALTH CONDITIONS AMONG ADULTS WITH DEVELOPMENTAL DISABILITIES IN PRIMARY CARE

SUZANNE MCDERMOTT, ROBERT R. MORAN
AND TAN PLATT

Nova Biomedical Books
New York

For permission to use material from this book please contact us:
Telephone 631-231-7269; Fax 631-231-8175
Web Site: http://www.novapublishers.com

NOTICE TO THE READER

The Publisher has taken reasonable care in the preparation of this book, but makes no expressed or implied warranty of any kind and assumes no responsibility for any errors or omissions. No liability is assumed for incidental or consequential damages in connection with or arising out of information contained in this book. The Publisher shall not be liable for any special, consequential, or exemplary damages resulting, in whole or in part, from the readers' use of, or reliance upon, this material.

Independent verification should be sought for any data, advice or recommendations contained in this book. In addition, no responsibility is assumed by the publisher for any injury and/or damage to persons or property arising from any methods, products, instructions, ideas or otherwise contained in this publication.

This publication is designed to provide accurate and authoritative information with regard to the subject matter covered herein. It is sold with the clear understanding that the Publisher is not engaged in rendering legal or any other professional services. If legal or any other expert assistance is required, the services of a competent person should be sought. FROM A DECLARATION OF PARTICIPANTS JOINTLY ADOPTED BY A COMMITTEE OF THE AMERICAN BAR ASSOCIATION AND A COMMITTEE OF PUBLISHERS.

Library of Congress Cataloging-in-Publication Data

McDermott, Suzanne, Ph. D.
  The epidemiology of common health conditions among adults with developmental disabilities in primary care / Suzanne McDermott and Tan Platt, Robert R. Moran, authors.
     p. ; cm.
Includes bibliographical references and index.
ISBN 978-1-60456-138-8 (hardcover)
1. Developmentally disabled--Health and hygiene--South Carolina. 2. Developmentally disabled--Medical care--South Carolina. 3. Primary care (Medicine)--South Carolina. I. Platt, Tan. II. Moran, Robert R. III. Title.
[DNLM: 1. Developmental Disabilities. 2. Adult. 3. Health Status. 4. Longitudinal Studies. 5. Primary Health Care. WM 140 M4776e 2007]
RC570.5.U6M33   2007
362.196'8--dc22   2007044356

Published by Nova Science Publishers, Inc. ✦ *New York*

Contents

Acknowledgement

This publication was supported by Cooperative Agreement Number R04/CCR418776 from the Centers for Disease Control and Prevention. Its contents are solely the responsibility of the authors and do not necessarily represent the official view of the Centers for Disease Control and Prevention.

This research is dedicated to adults with developmental disabilities whose health care is provided in primary care settings. The family physicians and nurse practitioners who provide the care should be commended for their years of caring service. We also thank the individual subjects in this study who have enriched our lives.

Preface

The purpose of this book is to provide evidence for physicians about the prevalence for a range of medical conditions by disability, from a primary care prospective.

Each chapter focuses on a secondary condition for which adults with DD are at increased risk, decreased risk, and the same risk as the general population. The incidence and prevalence of each of the secondary conditions is presented, and contrasted to the general population.The special challenges for diagnosis and treatment of the secondary condition is highlighted. Finally the book describes a case study that includes physical, social and emotional challenges and ways to accommodate these issues in a primary care practice.

Chapter I

Introduction

Purpose and Aim

This book is primarily written for researchers in the field of health and disability. The study results will also be informative for physicians, nurses, and providers of care for people with developmental disabilities (DD). We were inspired to write this book because there is insufficient information available about the natural history of aging for the ever increasing number of adults with developmental disabilities.

We are reporting on the results of a retrospective longitudinal study conducted in two family medicine centers where individuals with and without disabilities received primary care during the period 1993-2003. These findings come from a three year grant from the Centers for Disease Control and Prevention, Center for Birth Defects and Developmental Disabilities, to study the incidence and prevalence of common health conditions among adults with four domains of disability: developmental, mobility, psychiatric, and sensory. This book will report on a group of 694 adults with developmental disabilities and 1,809 comparison patients, all subgroups of the larger study. We used an average of ten years of follow-up data for the group with developmental disabilities and seven years of follow-up data for the adults without disability, resulting in over 19,500 person years of data on prevalence and incidence of common health conditions.

The larger study was a retrospective record review of 2,084 patients without disability and 1,451 patients with disability, including individuals with sensory disabilities (n=117), developmental disabilities (n=694), mobility-related disabilities (n=155) and psychiatric disabilities (n=485). In this book we will report on the two hypotheses for adults with developmental disabilities:

- Adults with developmental disabilities had higher prevalence of common health conditions, compared to adults without disability in the same practice.
- Adults with developmental disabilities who do not have the common health conditions when they enter the practices will have higher rates of onset compared to adults without disability in the same practice.

Background

There is a developing body of research that describes the onset of "secondary conditions" defined as "a preventable condition to which a person with a primary diagnosis is more susceptible and may include medical, physical, emotional, family, or community problems" (Lollar, 2001). However, the determination of "more susceptible" is often made through cross-sectional surveys to individuals about symptoms and diagnoses. This study was designed to use a longitudinal design to identify the onset of risk factors and conditions using a case group with disabilities and a comparison group from the same community who saw the same set of physicians for their primary care.

The concept of disability is slowly becoming a demographic descriptor instead of a synonym for poor health. The publication of Healthy People 2010 was the official beginning of the recognition of people with disability as a health disparity group. Disability joined gender, race/ethnicity, poverty, sexual orientation, income/education, and geographic location as the sixth Department of Health and Human Services recognized health disparity group. This is an important change in the conceptualization of disability since physicians and other practitioners need to address the presenting problem, within the context of disability, and not focus on the impairment when a primary care concern is presented. In addition, primary care providers also need to focus on health promotion, wellness, and prevention for these individuals as they move through the life span. For researchers the implications of disability as a demographic characteristic is equally important to recognize. Data on disability status should be collected prospectively in all population based research designs and analysis of results should include this characteristic in both descriptive and multivariable modeling.

The Centers for Disease Control and Prevention reports the prevalence of disability is approximately 20 percent of the US population. This estimate is based on responses to two Behavioral Risk Factor Surveillance System (BRFSS) questions that are asked on the telephone to a random sample of adults in all states. The two questions inquire about activity limitations and use of assistive devices:

- Are you limited in any way in any activities because of physical, mental, or emotional problems?
- Do you now have any health problem that requires you to use special equipment, such as a cane, a wheelchair, a special bed, or a special telephone? Include occasional use or use in certain circumstances (CDC, 2006).

The increasing prevalence rate for disability is in part the result of growth of the proportion of adults over the age of 65 years with age related conditions, the increase in life expectancy of survivors of birth defects, and the morbidity associated with childhood and young adult injuries and chronic illnesses. Disability is a consequence of a wide range of impairments and is an extremely heterogeneous demographic characteristic.

This book focuses on *developmental disabilities*, a subset of people with disability that contribute to a high proportion of disability years, since the onset is at birth or during childhood and their life expectancy for affected people now approaches the population average. The CDC defines developmental disabilities as "a diverse group of severe chronic conditions that are due to mental and/or physical impairments. People with developmental disabilities have problems with major life activities such as language, mobility, learning, self-help, and independent living. Developmental disabilities begin anytime during development up to 22 years of age and usually last throughout a person's lifetime" (CDC, 2004).

This book and the study we conducted is the result of efforts of professionals from complementary disciplines: a health services researcher and epidemiologist, a physician who provided care to the patients in the large urban practice, and a biostatistician. The expertise of the collaborators was needed to direct the complex and systematic review of medical records, develop a large relational data system, analyze the data, and interpret the results.

Conceptual Framework

Disability related mortality is replaced by morbidity as medical care improves for individuals with birth defects, injuries, and debilitating conditions. Primary care physicians need to know what to expect when a patient with a developmental disability joins their practice. For which conditions are individuals with developmental disabilities at increased risk? What conditions have no additional risk for individuals with developmental disabilities? For which conditions are individuals with developmental disabilities at reduced risk?

The challenge for researchers is to know more about adults with disabilities so they can be included in future research. In addition, researchers can observe how expected results are modified when people are observed longitudinally and when the comparison group includes people receiving the same care in the same setting. This study can help researchers understand the impact of unobserved confounding related to both community characteristics and medical practice patterns. We hope the study will provoke researchers to think about what questions remains unanswered and how to design a study in a primary care setting that can contribute to new knowledge.

The literature on the primary care needs of adults with developmental disabilities, of which the group with mental retardation (MR) is the largest, living in the community has grown substantially in the past two decade (Larson, et al, 1986; Rubin, et al, 1987; Ziring, et al, 1988; Day, et al, 1994; McDermott, et al, 1997; Kapell, et al, 1998; Smith, 2001; Phillips, et al, 2004; Tyler and Edman, 2004). A review of studies that include a comparison group, the patients with developmental disabilities had higher prevalence of epilepsy, diseases of the skin, and sensory loss (Kapell et al, 1998). We will review the literature on each of the common health conditions addressed in this book in terms of both adults with developmental disabilities and the general population.

Despite the significance of disability issues, the increasing prevalence of disability, and the annual disability related expenditures of over $200 billion, there are few studies of the risk for numerous common health conditions, comparing different disability groups in the same primary care setting (Albrecht, 2001). The purpose of this book is to provide evidence about the incidence and prevalence for a range of medical conditions for adults with developmental disabilities, from data collected over a ten-year period in primary care setting.

The use of two family physician practices as the setting for the study was an important decision. Since the largest proportion of ambulatory care services occurs in a physician office, the National Ambulatory Medical Care Survey (NAMCS) has been collecting data and reporting about the health care provided by office based physicians since 1973 (Advance Data No.374). There were on average 3.2 visits to US physician offices for every American in 2004 (NAMCS, 374) and 25% of these were to family medicine physicians. For the general population routine chronic problems accounted for one-third of the visits and the most frequent illness diagnoses for office visits were, in order of frequency, hypertension, cancers, acute upper respiratory infections, diabetes mellitus, rheumatoid arthritis, osteoarthritis and related disorders.

Implications of Our Study

We are able to describe the health and illness experience of adults with developmental disabilities compared to adults without disabilities who obtain their health care from the same providers and live in the same community. This reduces selection bias which plagues many studies when recruitment of the cases and comparison group come from different sites and communities. Our strategy reduces the problem of un-measurable variables (or residual confounding) as they relate to the local health care and community environment. The two medical practices serve a disproportionate proportion of people with Medicaid and Medicare insurance, thus from an income and age eligibility standpoint the case and the comparison group are comparable. The zip codes in which the cases and comparison group reside are the same.

The results of our research can be generalized to other family medicine practices, with a few cautions. The study was conducted in two counties in South Carolina. The large practice was in the state capital and this practice is a partnership between the University and a large public hospital. The second, small practice was in a rural county and the practice is a part of the same University network. The patient population served by these two practices has a higher rate of poverty compared to the general population. Thus, since a large proportion of people with developmental disabilities are poor we believe the comparison between the cases and the comparison group without disability was fair, but the generalizability to other more affluent communities should be made with caution. In addition, the two counties from which our patients were drawn are made up of primarily African-American and white residents, thus our results should not be applied to other racial and ethnic groups.

Organization of the Chapters

Each chapter is arranged in the same format. First we state the research questions. This is usually a question about the prevalence of the condition in adults with developmental disability compared to the comparison group and in most cases we also ask about incidence. For a few conditions we explored questions related to recovery (e.g. from obesity to normal weight) or onset given a pre-existing condition (e.g. diabetes onset given pre-existing obesity).

The second section is a review of the literature about the prevalence of the health condition in the general population. This is followed by the third section, a review of the literature about the prevalence among adults with developmental disabilities. The fourth section is a conceptual model for the question and it is intended to provide a context for the question within the domain of developmental disability. We explain why we think the health condition is different for people with developmental disabilities compared to the general population and we explore some related issues. The fifth section is a case study that was modified from actual individuals seen in one of the practices. The sixth section is our research findings where we present the results in both narrative and tabular form. The last two sections discuss the implications of our study findings for research and the implications for the case study, for those interested in clinical aspects of care.

The aim of this book is to inform researchers and clinicians about the health status of adults with developmental disabilities, stimulate additional questions about the health status of adults with developmental disabilities, and demonstrate a strategy to conduct research in a primary care setting.

References

Albrecht GL, Bury M. The political economy of the disability marketplace. In: GL Albecht, KD Seelman and M Bury (Eds.). *Handbook of Disability Studies*. Thousand Oaks California: Sage Publications, 2001 585–609.

Centers for Disease Control and Prevention. Developmental Disabilities [online]. Year [2004, October 29]. Available from: http://www.cdc.gov/ncbddd/dd/dd1/htm:

Centers for Disease Control and Prevention. *Disability and Health State Chartbook 2006: Profiles of Health for Adults with Disabilities*. Atlanta, GA.: Centers for Disease Control and Prevention; 2006.

Day K, Jancar J. Mental and physical health and aging in mental handicap: a review. *J. Intellect Disabil. Res.* 1994 38, 241–245.

Kapell D, Nightingale B, Rodriguez A, Lee JH, Zigman WB, Schupf N. Prevalence of chronic medical conditions in adults with mental retardation: comparison with the general population. *Ment. Retard.* 1998 36, 269–279.

Larson CP, Lapointe Y. The health status of mild to moderate intellectual handicapped adolescents. *J. Mental Defic. Res.* 1986 30,121–128.

Lollar, D.J. Public health trends in disability: past, present, and future. In: Albrecht, G.L., Seelman, K.D., Bury, M. (eds.), *Handbook of Disability Studies*. Thousand Oaks, CA: Sage Publications, Inc; 2001;754-771.

McDermott S, Platt T, Krishnaswami S. Are individuals with mental retardation at high risk for chronic disease?. *Fam. Med.* 1997 29, 429–434.

Phillips A, Morrison J, Davis RW. General practitioners' educational needs in intellectual disability health. *J. Intellect. Disabil. Res.* 2004 48, 142–149.

Rubin IL. Health care needs of adults with mental retardation. *Ment. Retard.* 1987 125, 201–206.

Smith, DS. Health care management of adults with Down syndrome. *American Family Physician*, 2001, 64, 6, 1031-8.

Tyler C, Edman JC. Down syndrome, Turner syndrome, and Klinefelter syndrome: primary care throughout the life span. *Prim. Care Clin. Office Pract.*, 2004, 31, 627-648.

Ziring PR, Kastner T, Friedman DL, et al. Provision of health care for persons with developmental disabilities living in the community. *JAMA* 1988 26,1439–1444.

Chapter II

Study Method

This study used a retrospective cohort design to analyze the incidence and prevalence of a range of common health conditions among adults with developmental disabilities and adults without disabilities receiving primary care in either a large urban family medicine center or a small rural practice. Both of the medical practices were staffed by family medicine physicians, nurses, and included medical student and residents.

Timeframe for the Study

The timeframe for the study included the period 1993-2003. Patients with an electronic medical record at one of the two study sites during this period were eligible for participation. Once an individual was selected for study participation we included information from both the computerized medical record and the companion paper records archived from earlier medical care, occasionally dating back to childhood. Thus, although the timeframe for data was typically eleven years or less, we had some participants with twenty years of data.

Study Participants

Patients with and without a primary disability were selected from a pool of over 58,000 individuals who received care at the study sites during the study period (1993 to 2003). There were 51,146 records at the urban site and 7,851 records at the rural site. Patients with a disability were identified as potential cases using the electronic medical records, using a search process that included both International Classification of Disease (ICD9) (World Health Organization, 2000) codes and the actual names and abbreviations for each of the disabilities.

The Case Group

We studied 694 individuals with a developmental disability (DD) including the following groups of adults:

- 54 with autism
- 58 with Down syndrome
- 163 with cerebral palsy (CP)
- 152 with mental retardation and psychiatric illness (MR and psychiatric illness)
- 267 with mental retardation (MR only).

The 694 unduplicated patients with a developmental disability were seen for a minimum of three visits at one of the family medicine sites during the period 1993-2003.

The Comparison Group

We had 1,809 comparison patients in the same medical practices. The comparison patients, without sensory, mobility, psychiatric, cognitive and developmental disabilities, were selected after all the patients with a disability were identified. Again we only selected individuals who were seen for a minimum of three visits at one of the family medicine sites during the period 1993-2003. We used age-group stratification for selection of the comparison group, basing the strata on the distribution of age in the cases with developmental disabilities. We used the same comparison group for all disability subgroups.

The comparison patients were proportionally matched in ten year increments based on age at entry into the practices. Thus, if 10% of the patients with developmental disabilities in our case group entered the practice between the ages 20-30 years, we selected patients without disabilities so that 10% also entered the practice during this same decade of life.

Participant Characteristics

Table 1 below shows the characteristics of the adults in our study. We had a mean of 10.3 years of follow-up for the participants with developmental disabilities and a mean of 7.1 years for the comparison group, without any lifelong disability, within the same practices.

We used the age at entry into the practice instead of date of birth since this minimized the bias of different ages under observation, between the case and comparison groups. It should be noted in Table 1 that the comparison patients were on average five years older than the patients with developmental disabilities and they had seven years of follow-up compared to ten years for the group with developmental disabilities. The age difference is a result of the age-group stratification being done when all the four disability groups (sensory, developmental, mobility, psychiatric) were included. The developmental disability group had the youngest mean age. The years of follow-up differed because the developmental disability group stayed on average three years longer in the two practices compared to the comparison group.

Table 1, Column 2 shows the characteristics of the 1,809 comparison patients selected from age-stratified groups of individuals in the practices who did not have a disability. Their average age at entry into the practices was 40 years and we had a little over seven years of follow-up. Fifty six percent were women which is typical of most medical practices.

The racial composition of the comparison patients was 50 percent African-American, 47 percent white, and 3 percent Asian, other or missing. It is important to note that 30 percent were current smokers at the time of the study and another 14 percent were past smokers.

Table 1, Columns 3 provides information about the developmental disability group as a whole, while the remaining columns show the variation between the sub-groups. There are notable differences in the entry age and in all cases the developmental disability sub-groups were younger than the comparison patients. The DD sub-groups all had longer follow-up time compared to the comparison group. The DD group was over 53% male and as expected the autism group was 78% male. The DD group had a higher proportion of white study participants, especially in the autism, Down syndrome, and cerebral palsy groups. The severity of the primary condition differed among the sub-groups with a higher proportion of moderate and severe cases for autism and Down syndrome. Diabetes and smoking was less prevalent in the developmental disability sub-groups compared to the patients without a disability, except in the group with MR and psychiatric illness where the proportion of current smokers was highest (35.5%).

The Practice Sites

The urban setting was a large practice with approximately 15 attending family medicine physicians, plus medical students, interns and residents in Family Medicine, and nurse practitioners involved in patient care. This practice is on the campus of a large public hospital with many outpatient and inpatient services in close proximity. The practice was established in the early 1970s as a residency practice of the community hospital and it has been affiliated with the University of South Carolina, School of Medicine since the school's inception in 1977. There are over 20,000 active patients in the practice each year and over 50,000 electronic medical records of those who have been patients during the study period of 1993-2003. The rural setting had one physician and one nurse practitioner as the primary providers although medical students and residents were also present. This practice is located next to a small rural hospital approximately 30 miles from the urban site.

Table 1. Characteristics of Patients by Group

	Comparison group without disability	With Developmental Disability	Autism	Down syndrome	Cerebral Palsy	MR with Psychiatric illness	MR Only
Sample Size (n)	1809	694	54	58	163	152	267
Entry Age (mean)	40.3	34.5	26.3	33.2	32.3	36.9	36.3
Folllow-up years (mean)	7.1	10.3	8.2	12.5	10.8	10.6	9.9
Person years	12,883	7,170	444	726	1,754	1,607	2,639
Gender (%)							
Male	43.6	53.2	77.8	58.6	45.4	48.7	54.3
Female	56.4	46.8	22.2	41.4	54.6	51.3	45.7
Race (%)							
White	46.9	59.8	70.4	74.1	65.0	49.3	57.3
African American	50.1	39.2	27.8	24.1	34.4	50.7	41.2
Other	2.3	0.4	1.8	0.0	0.6	0.0	0.4
Missing	0.7	0.6	0.0	1.8	0.0	0.0	1.1
Severity of Primary Disability (%)							
Mild	n/a	36.6	18.5	10.3	30.7	59.2	36.7
Moderate	n/a	26.5	72.2	13.8	34.4	13.8	22.5
Severe	n/a	36.9	9.3	75.9	34.9	27.0	40.8
Diabetes at entry	15.2	9.9	1.9	8.6	6.1	11.8	13.1
Smoking							
Current	29.9	17.4	3.7	10.3	6.1	35.5	18.4
Ever	13.8	4.8	0.0	0.0	1.8	4.6	8.6
None	56.3	77.8	96.3	89.7	92.1	59.9	73.0

Case Definitions for Disability Group

The term developmental disability has been used since the late 1960s to describe a group of conditions with early onset, long-term duration, developmental implications, and continuing service needs. The Rehabilitation Act Amendments of 1978 (PL 95-602) established the formal definition: "A severe, chronic disability of a person which (A) is attributable to a mental or physical impairment or combination of mental and physical impairments; (B) is manifested before the person attains the age twenty-two; (C) is likely to continue indefinitely; (D) results in substantial functional limitations in three or more of the following areas of major life activity: (i) self care, (ii) receptive and expressive language, (iii) learning, (iv) mobility, (v) self-direction, (vi) capacity for independent living, and (vii) economic self-sufficiency; and (E) reflects the individual's need for a combination and sequence of special, interdisciplinary, or generic services, individualized supports, or other forms of assistance that are of lifelong or extended duration and are individually planned and coordinated" (Ohio Legal Rights Service, 2007).

In our study we classified individuals based on the primary impairment underlying their disability: (1) autism, (2) Down syndrome, (3) cerebral palsy (CP) (4) MR with psychiatric illness (5) MR. Throughout the book the groups are mutually exclusive. We developed this classification system with the knowledge that the majority of adults with Down syndrome and many individuals with autism have mental retardation. We separated the group with Down syndrome from the others with MR because their medical profile is substantially different. In the cases with dual diagnoses of autism and mental retardation we used the primary diagnosis assigned by the physician. The MR group was split into two sub-groups based on the presence or absence of a major psychiatric diagnosis: schizophrenia or other psychosis. Both of the MR groups contain many individuals with unknown cause for the MR and some individuals with specific syndromes and diagnoses (excluding Down syndrome). The case definition of each of the developmental disabilities in our study is dependent on having the associated ICD9 code in the medical record or a text statement in the medical record that states the individual has the named disability. The specific disabilities are:

Autism: Autism is classified by the World Health Organization (WHO) and American Psychological Association as a developmental disability that results from a disorder of the human central nervous system (2000; 2004). The ICD9 code for autism is 299.0 (Medicode, 2001). Autism is diagnosed using specific criteria for impairments to social interaction, communication, interests, imagination and activities (World Health Organization, 2000) and on the basis of a triad of behavioral impairments or dysfunctions: 1. impaired social interaction, 2. impaired communication and 3. restricted and repetitive interests and activities (American Psychiatric Association, 1994). The co-occurrence of mental retardation with autism is reported to be 50-60% although recent reviews of the evidence indicates the proportion of children with both MR and autism is probably lower than previously thought. (Bolte, Poustka, 2002; Volkmar et al., 2004).

Down syndrome: Down syndrome is also described as Trisomy 21 and it is assigned the ICD9 code 758.0 (Medicode, 2001). Down syndrome is the most prevalent known genetic cause of mental retardation and is caused by a translocation of all or major parts of chromosome 21 (Roizen, Patterson, 2003). Individuals with Down syndrome can exhibit all levels of cognitive function from mild to profound mental retardation and they have distinct dysmorphic features.

Cerebral Palsy: Cerebral palsy is a term used to describe a group of chronic conditions affecting body movements and muscle coordination. It is assigned ICD9 code of 343 (Medicode, 2001). "The term cerebral palsy refers to any one of a number of neurological disorders that appear in infancy or early childhood and permanently affect body movement and muscle coordination but don't worsen over time. Even though cerebral palsy affects muscle movement, it isn't caused by problems in the muscles or nerves. It is caused by abnormalities in parts of the brain that control muscle movements. The majority of children with cerebral palsy are born with it, although it may not be detected until months or years later. The early signs of cerebral palsy usually appear before a child reaches 3 years of age. The most common are a lack of muscle coordination when performing voluntary movements (ataxia); stiff or tight muscles and exaggerated reflexes (spasticity); walking with one foot or leg dragging; walking on the toes, a crouched gait, or a "scissored" gait; and muscle tone that is either too stiff or too floppy." (National Institute of Neurological Disorders and Stroke, 2007). Depending on which areas of the brain have been damaged, one or more of the following may occur: muscle tightness or spasm, involuntary movement, disturbance in gait and mobility, abnormal sensation and perception, impairment of sight, hearing or speech, or seizures. CP is a clinical diagnosis; no laboratory test or tissue histology defines its presence or absence. In addition, despite the usefulness of CT and MRI scanning, no single neuro-imaging pattern encompasses the diagnostic findings that are possible in CP.

Mental Retardation: Mental retardation is a disability characterized by significant limitations both in intellectual functioning and in adaptive behavior as expressed in conceptual, social, and practical adaptive skills. This disability originates before age 18 and the ICD9 codes are 317, 318 and 319 (Medicode, 2001). Assignment of one of these three ICD9 codes is based on a combination of IQ score and adaptive behavior. Mental Retardation is characterized by limitations in present functioning and must be considered within the context of community environments typical of the individual's age peers and culture. Adaptive behavior is the collection of conceptual, social, and practical skills that people have learned so they can function in their everyday lives. Significant limitations in adaptive behavior impact a person's daily life and affect the ability to respond to a particular situation or to the environment. Limitations in adaptive behavior can be determined by using standardized tests that are normed on the general population including people with disabilities and people without disabilities. On these standardized measures, significant limitations in adaptive behavior are operationally defined as performance that is at least two standard deviations below the mean of either (a) one of the following three types of adaptive behavior: conceptual, social, or practical, or (b) an overall score on a standardized measure of conceptual, social, and practical skills (AAIDD, 2001).

Mental Retardation with Psychiatric Illness: These individuals have characteristics that meet the case definition for MR described above and have a diagnosis of schizophrenia (ICD9 295) or bipolar disorder or other psychotic condition (ICD9 296) (Medicode, 2001). These psychiatric conditions are often grouped into a category of severe mental illness with a prevalence of approximately three percent of the US population (USDHHS, 1999). The prevalence of psychiatric illness among adults with mental retardation is substantially higher. There is great variability in the estimated dual diagnosis of mental retardation and psychiatric illness ranging from 10-80 percent depending on the diagnostic criteria used, the sample of patients surveyed, the level of MR, and the way the psychiatric evaluation was conducted (Matson and Laud, 2007). The combination of ICD9 codes required for classification of individuals into this group are: ICD9 (317 or 319 or 319) and ICD9 (295 or 296) (Medicode, 2001).

Table 2 summarizes the conditions included in our case group and their ICD9 codes.

Table 2. Primary Disabling Conditions and ICD9 Codes

Condition, Abbreviation, and Search Terms	ICD9 code
Primary disabilities	
*Affectives Psychoses: Bipolar, manic-depressive, depressive psychoses	296
Autism or Pervasive Developmental Disability (PDD)	299
Cerebral Palsy (CP)	343
Translocation Down syndrome (DS) or Trisomy 21	758
Mental Retardation (MR)	317, 318, 319
*Schizophrenia	295

*Affective psychoses and schizophrenia were only used in combination with an ICD9 code for MR of 317, 318 or 319 to define a subgroup with MR and psychiatric illness.

Identifying Common Health Conditions

The common health conditions included in this study were selected from a review of the literature on office-based medical practices, ambulatory care visits, and leading causes of death in the US. Cardiovascular disease is the leading cause of death and accounts for a substantial proportion of ambulatory care visits. We included congestive heart failure, coronary artery disease, and hypertension in our list of conditions. We included the two most prevalent chronic respiratory conditions: asthma and chronic obstructive pulmonary disease. Likewise diabetes and dementia are among the top ten leading causes of death in the US. Finally, we included depression the most prevalent psychiatric diagnosis in primary care. We also included obesity in our study since is one of the top risk factors for disease. We did not include cancer, injuries, influenza, and septicemia in this study even though these are listed among the top ten causes of death in the US. We made the decision to exclude cancer since we anticipated insufficient numbers of each type of cancer, given our sample size and the expected prevalence. We did not include injuries, influenza, and septicemia since we focused on chronic conditions and we categorized these conditions as acute conditions. Lastly, we included seizure as a common health condition since this is the case for adults with developmental disabilities, although it is not the case for the general population.

The eleven common health conditions we studied and their associated ICD9 codes are shown in Table 3. We also studied death as our twelfth outcome.

Table 3. Common Health Conditions

Common Health Conditions	ICD9 code
Asthma	493
Chronic Obstructive Pulmonary Disease (COPD)	490-492, 494-496
Congestive Heart Failure (CHF)	428
Coronary Artery Disease (CAD)	413, 414
Dementia	290, 331
Depression	300, 311, 309
Diabetes (DM, Type 1, Type 2)	250
Epilepsy	345, 780.39
Hypertension (HTN, HBP)	401
Obesity	278

We coded the common health conditions as present based on either the inclusion of the diagnosis, abbreviation, or ICD9 code in the medical record problem list or in the medical note, if it was stated in the affirmative as a diagnosis. We also used the medication lists and the diagnostic test reports to supplement our condition finding. When medications for a specific condition were prescribed we double checked the record to determine if their use was for the diagnosis of interest. Likewise we looked at medical test results and double checked the record to determine if a diagnosis had been made. All medical records, including paper and electronic documents, were read to identify these diagnoses. In all cases where the medical coders were uncertain about the diagnosis, the case was reviewed at the weekly study meeting, and the Medical Director made a determination about the diagnosis. Death was defined only by finding a study participant in the death file from the National Death Registry.

We used the criteria for disease and condition diagnosis that was endorsed by Evidence Based Practice guidelines during the time when the diagnosis was made. Thus, if the standard for diabetes diagnosis changed in 2004, after the study period, we applied the diagnostic standard that was used during the 1990-2003 period. If the standard changed within our study interval we used the standard that was accepted at the time the actual diagnosis was made. Therefore, all cases of diabetes in this study were not based on the same criterion; instead they reflect the practice guidelines during our study interval.

Data on Independent Variables

The following independent variables were evaluated: age, race, smoking status, gender, and medical practice site. We also included presence of a diagnosis of diabetes and the starting BMI for some of the conditions. For example we controlled for obesity in those with diabetes and later stratified by this effect modifier. We used diabetes as an independent variable when we studied obesity and congestive heart failure.

For the sub-groups with developmental disability we added the level of MR and the residence type. The most restrictive environment (MRE) included Community Training Homes and ICF-MR (Intermediate Care Facilities for Persons with MR). Community Training homes are small home-like environments under the supervision of a qualified and trained caregiver. Personalized care, supervision and individualized training are provided for no more than three individuals living in a home. Caregivers are either trained private citizens who provide care in their own homes (CTH I), or employees who provide care in a home that is owned or rented by the provider organization (CTH II). Community Residential Care Facilities (CRCF) and ICF-MR are structured residential settings with 24-hour supervision and health and rehabilitative services. ICF-MR facilities usually provide housing for 8-12 individuals who need the most intense physical and psychiatric supports.

The Least Restrictive Environment (LRE) included family home, private boarding home, supervised apartment living, and supervised living in a private home contracted through the state disability agency. Supervised living programs serve adults capable of a significant degree of independence. Adults may live in apartments, duplexes or other housing and supervision and support services are provided to meet individual needs. Supervised living programs (SLP-1 and SLP-2) resemble single-family homes in local neighborhoods. They provide 24-hour care, supervision, counseling, recreation and other activities. For addition detail about residential types see Appendix A.

The dichotomous variables that were included as independent variables were: race (non-white, white), gender (male, female), smoking status (smoked cigarettes at some time during the years in the practice- yes, no), medical practice site (urban, rural), and residence (most restrictive environment (MRE)/ least restrictive environment (LRE)). The developmental disability was a categorical variable with three levels: mild, moderate and severe. The continuous independent variables were age at entry into the family medicine practices, body mass index (BMI), and number of years of follow-up.

Data Collection and Analysis

Data were collected by two full time medical record abstracters and a cadre of part-time coders, under the regular supervision of the study physician. The information abstracted included all notations and dates of physical findings, vital signs, diagnoses, medical procedures, laboratory and diagnostic test results, and medication orders from physician dictated progress notes, problem lists, medication files, and consultation notes in individual records.

Data were analyzed using the SAS statistical package. Initially we divided the individuals with developmental disabilities into their primary diagnostic group and looked at the distributions of the independent variables for each group. Differences between diagnostic groups in the continuous variables such as age at entry into the practice were analyzed using t-tests and differences in categorical variables such as gender and race were analyzed using the X^2 test. We used these methods to calculate group differences in the demographic and lifestyle characteristics which were available in the medical records. Prevalence of each medical condition was analyzed for each disability category using the number of individuals with the condition in the numerator and the number of individuals with the primary disabling condition in the denominator.

Logistic regression was used to assess the unadjusted odds ratios for each condition. We then calculated the *adjusted odds ratio* controlling for age, race, gender, practice location, starting BMI, tobacco use, and severity of the primary disability. Survival analysis, using Cox proportional hazards, modeled the onset of the conditions in patients with and without disability. The years when patients were seen by providers in the practice were summed and used as patient years. Only patients without the secondary medical condition when they entered the practice were included in the individual medical condition survival analysis, so onset could be observed. Again the same potentially confounding variables (race, gender, practice location, starting BMI, diabetes, tobacco use, and severity of the primary disability) were entered into all of the hazard functions. The final hazard functions were models that included the disability status and the confounders that were associated with the onset of each of the health conditions.

References

American Association of Mental Retardation. *Frequently Asked Questions About Mental Retardation* [online]. Year [2007, February 13]. Available from: http://www.aamr.org/Policies/faq_mental_retardation.shtml:

American Psychiatric Association. *Diagnostic and Statistical Manual of Mental Disorders.* Fourth edition. Washington, DC: American Psychiatric Association; 1994.

Bolte, S. and Poustka, F. (2002). The relation between general cognitive level and adaptive behavior domains in individuals with autism with and without co-morbid mental retardation. *Child Psychiatry and Human Development*, 2002 33, 165-72.

Matson JL, Laud, RB. Assessment and treatment psychopathology among people with developmental delay. In: Jacobson JW, Mulick JA, and Rojahn, J. (2007) *Handbook of intellectual and developmental disabilities.* Springer Press, NY, 507-39.

Medicode. *ICD-9-CM Professional For Physicians*, Volumes 1 and 2. Sixth edition. West Valley City, UT: Medicode ingenix companies; 2001.

National Institute of Neurological Disorders and Stroke. *What is Cerebral Palsy.* [online] 2007, June 20. Available from: http://www.ninds.nih.gov/disorders/cerebral_palsy/cerebral_palsy.htm:

Ohio Legal Rights Service. *U.S. Code Definition of Developmental Disability* [online]. 2007, March 12. Available from:http://olrs.ohio.gov/asp/olrs_DD_defineTXT.asp:

Roisen NJ, Patterson D., Down syndrome. *Lancet,* 2003, 361 (9365), 1281-9.

U.S. Department of Health and Human Services. *Mental Health: A Report of the Surgeon General-Executive Summary* [online]. Year [2007, February 12]. Available from: http://www.surgeongeneral.gov/library/mentalhealth/pdfs/ExSummary-Final.pdf:

Volkmar FR, Lord C, Bailey A, et al. Autism and pervasive developmental disorders. *J. Child Psychol. Psychiatry*, 2004 45, 135-70.

World Health Organization. *International Statistical Classification of Diseases.* 9th ed. Geneva, Switzerland, 2000.

Chapter III

Obesity

The Research Questions: (1) What is the prevalence of obesity in adults with developmental disabilities and how does this compare to adults without a disability, after controlling for known risk factors? (2) For those adults who are not obese when they enter the family medicine study sites, are there differences in the proportion of people who become obese among the impairment groups compared to those without a disability? (3) For those adults who are obese when they enter the family medicine study sites, are there different proportions of people who return to normal weight among the impairment groups compared to those without a disability?

Definition of Obesity and Prevalence in the General Population: Obesity is defined by the National Institute of Health as having a high amount of body fat. A person is considered obese if he or she has a body mass index (BMI) of 30 kg/m2 or greater (National Institute of Diabetes, Digestive, and Kidney Diseases, 2007). Body Mass Index has become the standard for relating adult weight to height in order to make an assessment of appropriate weight status. According to most experts a BMI (weight/height squared) between 18.5 and 25 is normal, 25-29 is overweight, a BMI greater than 30 is obese, and a BMI greater than 40 is morbid obesity.

The US prevalence of obesity (BMI$\geq$30) in 2000 was 30.9% (Flegal et al, 2002). The US Surgeon General report of 2001 described obesity as an epidemic in the US in all age groups, racial and ethnic groups, and both genders. (US Department of Health and Human Services et al, 2001). According to self-reported measures of height and weight, obesity (BMI $\geq$ 30) has been increasing in every State in the Nation.

Based on clinical height and weight measurements during the period 2003-2004 in the National Health and Nutrition Examination Survey (NHANES), 31.1 percent of U.S. men and 33.2 percent of women were obese. Obesity had statistically significantly increased for men between 1999-2000 (from 27.5%) but it did not significantly increase for women during this same period adults aged 20 to 74 years are overweight (BMI 25 to 29.9), and an additional 27 percent are obese (BMI $\geq$ 30) (Flegal, Carroll, Ogden, and Johnson et al, 2002).

Literature Review of Obesity in Adults with Developmental Disability: Obesity has been reported to be more prevalent among individuals with MR compared to the general population, with reports of prevalence as high as 30-50 percent (Rubin, Rimmer, Chicoine, Braddock, and McGuire, et al, 1998; Harris et al, 2003; Rimmer and Wang, 2005; Yamaki, 2005). The National Health Interview Survey was used to estimate the prevalence of obesity among adults with developmental disabilities compared to the general population living in the community during the year 2000 and the prevalence of obesity for adults with developmental disability was 34.6%, this was statistically significantly higher than obesity among adults without self-reported developmental disability (Yamaki et al, 2005).

Several cross sectional studies of people with MR that have found that the rates of obesity are higher in females (Rimmer, Braddock, and Fujiura et al, 1993), in those with mild MR , those living in the least restrictive environments, including family homes and in apartments without extensive supervision in the community (Rimmer, Braddock, and Fujiura et al, 1993; Fox and Rotatori et al, 1982; Rimmer, Braddock, and Marks et al, 1995) , and those living in the US (Harris et al, 2003). Also, persons with Down syndrome have been reported to be 1.3 – 1.8 times more likely to be obese compared to other individuals with MR (Prasher et al, 1995; Fujiura, Fitzsimons, and Marks et al, 1997; Rubin, Rimmer, Chicoine, Braddock, and McGuire et al, 1998; Bell and Bhate et al, 1992).

The association of Down syndrome and obesity has been studied by a number of researchers. Rimmer and Wang (2005) evaluated 91 adults with other causes of mental retardation and 58 adults with Down syndrome and found 60.4% of those with MR and 70.7% of those with Down syndrome were obese. A case-control study was conducted in the United Kingdom comparing the BMI for people with Down syndrome and age, gender, and residential type matched controls. For the 247 matched pairs women with Down syndrome had higher BMI than the controls. Men with Down syndrome were more likely to be in the overweight category than their matched pairs but were less likely to be obese (OR 0.85) (Melville, Cooper, McGrother, Thorp, and Collacott, et al, 2005).

What is the Conceptual Framework for this question?: The prevalence of obesity among adults with mental retardation and the impact on their lives is thought to be even greater than the general population. "The disadvantages associated with impaired cognitive function are compounded when an individual is perceived to be unattractive, have lower stamina, and higher risk for illness, traits often associated with obesity and mental retardation" (Moran, Drane, McDermott, Dasari, Scurry, and Platt et al, 2005). Adults with developmental disabilities often lead restricted lives, with limitations based on both their own challenges and those of their caregivers. As an outcome of efforts to focus on safety, many caregivers have limited activity and others have inadvertently encouraged sedentary lifestyle because of their own preferences. In addition, to provide rewards for accomplishments some caregivers have used food treats. The combination of these forces, along with some intrinsic factors related to short stature and low muscle tone for some known causes of MR can increase the likelihood of obesity.

Case Study: CJ was 32 years old when he was admitted from his parent's home to the local Intermediate Care Facility for adults with mental retardation (ICF-MR). Dr. A. is the

Medical Director for the community program that manages the home. CJ had cerebral palsy with spastic quadriplegia (ICD9 code 343.2) and moderate MR (ICD9 318.0) since birth and he uses a wheelchair for mobility. At the time of his physical examination, required before admission to the ICF-MR, CJ was 66 inches tall and weighed 195 pounds, resulting in a BMI of 31.6. In addition, he was diagnosed with hypertension (ICD9 401.9) and was on antihypertensive medications: hydrochlorothiazide (Microzide), lisinopril (Prinivil) and nifedipine (Procardia). He also had borderline elevated glucose. Dr. A. noted through a review of old records that CJ's condition was complicated by a seizure disorder (ICD9 345.10) and chronic depression (ICD9 311). He had previously lived in his parent's home but reports indicate for the previous ten years he interacted little in his home community.

At the time of his physical examination, Dr. A. ordered medications for blood pressure, epilepsy, and depression, weekly blood pressure and weight monitoring, and a 2000 calorie low fat diet. Soon after arrival in the ICF-MR CJ was started on the low calorie diet that was designed by the disability service agency dietician. The diet was used by staff to prepare his meals and snacks and over the next 3 years CJ lost 38 pounds. At a weight of 157 lbs and a BMI of 25 Dr. A. was able to eliminate one of his blood pressure medications, the depression medication, and CJ's serum glucose returned to normal. In addition a motorized wheelchair was obtained and CJ progressed in learning independent living skills that showed he was capable of living in a less supervised setting. He moved to a community training home (CTH) where he assumed more independence and CJ began to do his own shopping with minimal assistance.

Over the next 5 years Dr. A. observed CJ's weight gradually increased to 178 lbs or a BMI of 28.8 where it has stabilized. About twice or three times a year Dr. A. brings up issues related to diet including 5 a day fruit and vegetable intake and limiting calories and high fat foods. CJ's glucose has remained controlled, but he is once again taking 3 antihypertensive medications. He has been able to maintain this weight for the past 10 years.

Our Research Findings: BMI was recorded as a continuous variable at each clinic visit and then categorized into normal (<25), overweight (25-29), obese (30-39), morbid obesity (40 or higher).

This study was conducted in South Carolina, where obesity is a substantial problem. Our study results indicate that 46.1 percent of the comparison group, without disabilities, had a BMI greater than 30 at some time in their adult life. Overall, the developmental disability subgroup with the highest risk for ever being categorized as obese were those with Down syndrome, with 62 percent having a BMI greater than 30 at some time in their adult life. The DD group with the lowest risk of being categorized as obese were those with cerebral palsy, with 21 percent having a BMI over 30 recorded at some time during their medical care at one of the two practice sites (Moran, Drane, McDermott, Dasari, Scurry, and Platt et al, 2005). These results are shown in Table 1.

It is well known that there is a strong influence of age on BMI. We found the prevalence of obesity for adults with Down syndrome was 15.6% during the decade of age 20-30 and there was a steadily increasing proportion in each consecutive decade. There were significant differences in the proportion with obesity based on residential type and presence or absence of mental illness for those with mental retardation. During the decades of 30-40 and 40-50 a significantly greater proportion of individuals were obese if they lived in least restrictive environments (p<0.05) compared to most restrictive environments. During the decades of age 20-30, 30-40, and 40-50 the proportion of individuals with obesity was significantly higher among individuals with MR and a diagnosis of severe mental illness (SMI) compared to patients with MR without SMI (p<=0.05) (Moran, Drane, McDermott, Dasari, Scurry, and Platt et al, 2005).

The prevalence of obesity among those with MR, for each decade between age 20 and 60 and older is shown in Table 2. The percent of patients without disability, with a BMI 30 or greater was lowest (36.5%) for the decade of 20-30 years and highest (42.6%) for the decade 40-50 years. The proportion of mild MR patients with obesity was very similar to obesity proportion for the group without disability. Patients with severe MR had substantially lower rates of obesity, compared to the other groups, although they also had an upward trend in prevalence rates, to a high of 37.6% by age-group 50-60 years (Moran, Drane, McDermott, Dasari, Scurry, and Platt et al, 2005).

We used logistic regression to estimate the risk for ever having obesity for patients with DD compared to patients without any disability, controlling for gender, body mass index, age and tobacco use. The risk factors that were associated with increased risk were being female (Odds Ratio 1.65, p=0.001) and each year of age was associated with a protective effect (Odds Ratio 0.99, p=0.045). Past history of diabetes was a strong predictor of obesity with OR = 3.36 (p=0.001). African Americans were much more likely compared to whites to be obese with (Odds Ratio 1.56, p=0.001).

When we explored the likelihood of obesity among the different sub-groups with developmental disability compared to those without a disability we found the adults with cerebral palsy were statistically significantly less likely to be obese (Adjusted Odds Ratio 0.32, 95% Confidence Interval 0.21-0.48, p=0.001) and the adults with Down syndrome were statistically significantly more likely to be obese (Adjusted Odds Ratio 2.45, 95% Confidence Interval 1.40-4.29, p=0.002). These results are shown in Table 3.

We also explored the likelihood of developing obesity among those who entered the medical practices in the normal body mass index range. We found the risk of developing obesity was statistically significantly lower for those with cerebral palsy (Hazard Ratio 0.77, p=0.024), compared to the patients without disabilities. We also found autism (HR 2.27, p=0.001) and Down syndrome (HR 1.63, p=0.001) to be statistically significantly higher. There was no statistically significant difference in the risk for onset of obesity for those with MR with psychiatric illness or MR only, after controlling for the known risk factors (Table 4).

Table 1. Prevalence of Obesity among adults without disability and those with developmental disability, by sub-group and risk factors

Prevalence Obese	Without disability	All DD	Autism	Down syndrome	Cerebral Palsy	MR with Psychiatric Illness	Mental Retardation
Number in group	1809	694	54	58	163	152	267
Ever Obese	46.1	39.8	40.7	62.1	20.9	46.1	42.7
Gender							
Male	38.9	35.0	40.5	55.9	16.2	35.1	37.9
Female	51.7	45.2	41.7	70.8	24.7	56.4	48.4
Race							
White	37.6	39.8	42.1	65.1	21.7	44.0	42.5
African American	55.2	40.4	40.0	57.1	19.6	48.1	43.6
Other	29.3	0.0	0.0	0.0	0.0	0.0	0.0
Severity of Primary Disability							
Mild	n/a	n/a	50.0	83.3	34.0	56.7	52.0
Moderate	n/a	n/a	43.6	50.0	19.6	33.3	53.3
Severe	n/a	n/a	0.0	61.4	10.5	29.3	28.4
Residential Type							
Least Restrictive Environment	n/a	52.7	100.0	58.3	30.0	69.6	50.0
Most Restrictive Environment	n/a	33.0	31.3	43.8	17.2	38.9	40.0

Table 2. Proportion of adults with mental retardation, with obesity during decades of adult life

Person years	20 - 29	%	30-40	%	40-50	%	50-60	%	60+	%
Group										
Comparison	2,676	36.5	3,319	36.7	2,772	42.6	1,952	34.3	703	43.5
Developmental Disability	3,290	23.5	1,547	26.4	1,016	29.1	539	33.0	229	32.4
Autism	288	24.2	49	12.1	38	47.8	11	19.5	-	n/a
Down syndrome	420	25.9	141	30.5	86	36.5	50	38.8	-	n/a
Cerebral Palsy	878	12.5	325	10.0	194	31.1	95	20.0	40	0.0
MR with psychiatric illness	666	35.5	414	34.6	279	31.4	119	35.2	59	20.4
MR Only	1,038	24.0	618	29.7	418	23.4	264	36.2	130	47.7
Gender										
Male	1,884	32.3	1,709	32.0	989	64.1	796	41.8	263	38.9
Female	4,215	27.1	3,241	33.3	2,311	36.5	1,643	31.3	552	51.0
Race										
White	3,007	22.5	2,320	24.7	2,168	33.4	1,407	29.7	506	31.3
African-American	2,889	37.1	2,425	43.1	1,546	46.9	1,061	39.8	419	52.6
Other	40	10.2	102	8.0	64	41.9	22	38.1	4	13.5
Residence										
Least Restrictive Environment	685	31.4	280	30.3	123	32.9	78	34.7	6	0.0
Most Restrictive Environment	967	17.2	258	11.2	309	26.6	120	27.9	65	23.2
MR Severity										
Mild	1,383	37.3	657	34.2	362	28.0	208	33.8	107	44.1
Severe	1,619	11.4	753	166.0	531	24.2	258	37.6	89	22.9

Table 3. Logistic Regression Results for Risk of having obesity, by group adjusting for known risk factors

Groups	n	Prev.	Adjusted Odds Ratio	Lower Confidence Interval	Upper Confidence Interval	P-Value
Comparison	1809	46.1	1.00			
Autism	54	40.7	1.09	0.61	1.93	0.778
Cerebral Palsy	163	20.9	**0.32**	**0.21**	**0.48**	**0.001**
Down syndrome	58	62.1	**2.45**	**1.40**	**4.29**	**0.002**
MR with Psychiatric Illness	152	46.1	1.05	0.74	1.48	0.777
MR Only	267	42.7	0.93	0.71	1.22	0.585

* adjusted for medical site, gender, age, diabetes, and tobacco use.
Bold indicates statistically significant results.

Table 4. Survival Analysis* for Risk of Developing Obesity if entering the practice without obesity, by group

Groups	N	Hazard Ratio	P-Value
Comparison	1386		
Autism	46	**2.27**	**0.001**
Cerebral Palsy	150	**0.77**	**0.024**
Down syndrome	47	**1.63**	**0.001**
MR with Psychiatric Illness	117	1.18	0.081
MR Only	223	0.98	0.793

* controlling for medical site, age, gender, race, diabetes, current smoker.
Bold indicates statistically significant results.

Figure 1 shows the prevalence of obesity for patients with mental retardation compared to comparison patients in the same medical practices.

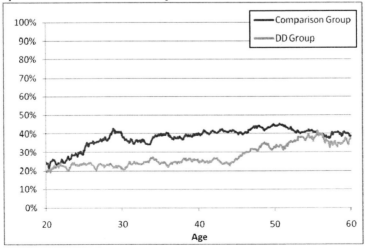

Figure 1. Proportion Patients with All Developmental Disabilities (DD) and Comparison Patients with BMI $\geq$ 30, by ages 20-60 years.

It is noteworthy that there is no statistically significant difference between the patients without disability and those with disability for ever having obesity and having obesity at each age. We then examined the impact of severity of disability and the risk for disability. Figure 2 shows the statistically significant difference between the patients with severe MR compared to those without disability between ages 20-30 (p=0.005), 30-40 years and 40-50 years (p<0.0001) (Moran, Drane, McDermott, Dasari, Scurry, and Platt et al, 2005).

In addition, we looked at the type of residential setting to see if a less restrictive environment, with fewer controls on the decisions made by the individual with DD, to see if there was a higher ratio of obesity compared to those living in more restrictive environments. Figure 3 shows the impact of residential type on obesity. Patients, age 30-40 years and those 40-50 years, who live in a more restrictive environment are statistically significantly less likely to be obese compared to those living in less restrictive environments (Moran, Drane, McDermott, Dasari, Scurry, and Platt et al, 2005).

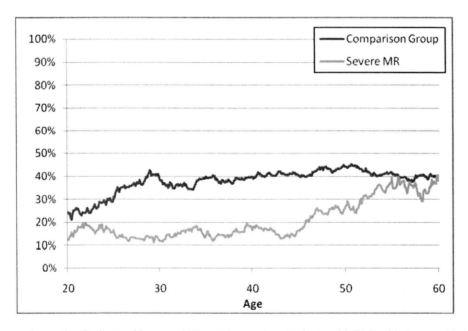

Figure 2. Proportion Patients with severe MR and Comparison Patients with BMI≥30, by ages 20-60 years.

Finally, we used survival analysis to determine if a different proportion of adults with obesity and disabilities compared to those with obesity but no disability, reverted to normal weight after entering the Family Medicine sites with obesity. Table 5 shows that the groups with cerebral palsy, Down syndrome, and both MR groups were more likely to lose weight compared to those without disability after entering care at one of the Family Medicine sites and the results were statistically significant.

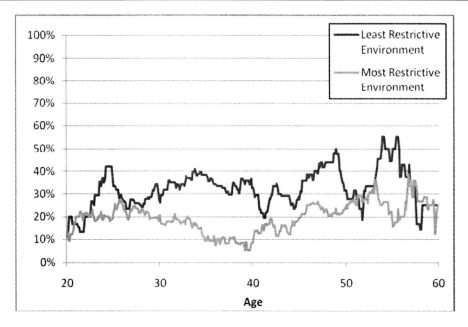

Figure 3. Patients with MR who had obesity, for each age, by level of residence.

Table 5. Survival Analysis* for Risk of becoming normal weight if entering the practice with obesity, by group

Groups	N	Hazard Ratio	P-Value
Comparison	834		
Autism	22	2.23	0.431
Cerebral Palsy	34	**6.98**	**0.001**
Down syndrome	36	**3.00**	**0.007**
MR with Psychiatric Illness	70	**4.76**	**0.001**
MR Only	114	**3.39**	**0.001**

* adjusted for medical site, gender, age, diabetes, and tobacco use.
Bold indicates statistically significant results.

Implications from our study findings: Our most important finding was that people with DD were more likely than the comparison group to lose weight once they reached obesity (Figure 5). We also found that among individuals with MR those living in the most restrictive environment had lower prevalence rates of obesity between the ages of 30 and 50 years. After age 50, the adults with MR living in more restrictive environments caught up to the higher rates of obesity among those in less restrictive environments and there was no significant difference between the two groups. This study's findings did not differ from earlier reports that women, African Americans, smokers, patients with Down syndrome, and those living in community settings had higher rates of obesity compared to their counterparts: males, whites, patients with other types of MR, and those living in more restrictive environments (Moran, Drane, McDermott, Dasari, Scurry and Platt et al, 2005).

It is important to note we did not find that patients with mild MR had higher rates of obesity compared to individuals without disability. And patients with severe MR had significantly lower prevalence of obesity compared to patients without disability through age 50 years. The likely reasons we found similar obesity prevalence between patients with mild MR and patients without disability was based on the practices where recruitment occurred. In a 1997 cross sectional analysis of one of the practices used in this study, the prevalence of obesity was lower in a group of patients with MR compared to other Medicaid insured patients in the same medical practice (McDermott, Platt, Krishnaswami, 1997). Thus, when a comparison is made within patients with the same insurance status, the results are different from studies in the literature reports comparisons between people with MR and patients with private insurance" (Moran, Drane, McDermott, Dasari, Scurry, and Platt et al, 2005).

The most encouraging finding of our study was weight loss during adult years is possible for people with developmental disabilities. The individuals with cerebral palsy, Down syndrome, and the two groups with mental retardation who entered the practice with obesity were statistically significantly more likely to lose weight compared to those without disability. The Hazard Rates indicate those with developmental disabilities with obesity were 2-7 times more likely to return to normal weight compared to the comparison group. Unless physicians understand the pattern of obesity prevalence and the evidence that people can move out of the obese state, concern about diet and exercise might recede from the forefront of physician-patient counseling sessions.

Since obesity is a substantial cardiovascular health risk and a clear impediment to community participation its importance should not be overlooked by health care providers, community service professionals, families and individuals with disabilities. Obesity can be prevented or treated if individuals and families recognize the health and lifestyle benefits of maintaining healthy weights. There is a popular view that obesity is a chronic condition. Our evidence suggests weight is a dynamic state with movement out of obesity and this is something all physicians should understand and encourage (Moran, Drane, McDermott, Dasari, Scurry, and Platt et al, 2005).

Implications for Case Study: CJ illustrates clearly the findings of the study. He came into Dr. A's practice with a BMI that classified him as obese. Not unexpectedly he was able to lose a significant amount of weight in a restrictive living environment. However, when he moved to a less restricted living situation and he started making choices for himself, he gained weight. Dr. A. provided ongoing instruction about diet for CJ and his caregivers using motivational interviewing skills to assess barriers and concerns. During most of CJ's visits, Dr. A. used a CPT code of 99214 to bill Medicaid since counseling was an important component of his care. CJ illustrates that a patient with significant cognitive and physical disabilities can have success in weight management and maintain it over many years with minimal physician intervention. The burden of obesity is multifaceted since it has the potential to impact health, social life, employment and an individual's general sense of well-being. Dr. A. understands that obesity is both preventable and treatable through lifestyle modification, including exercise and diet. So despite public and medical skepticism about the efficacy of weight loss approaches Dr. A's successfully worked with CJ to lose and maintain a healthy BMI.

References

Allison, DB; Gomez, JE; Heshka, S. Decreased resting metabolic rate among persons with Down syndrome. *Int. J. Obes. Relat. Metab. Disord.*, 1995 19, 858–861.

Flegal, KM; Carroll, MD; Ogden, CL. Prevalence and trends in obesity among US adults 1999-2000. *JAMA,* 2002 288, 1723-27.

Fujiura, GT; Fitzsimons, N; Marks B. Predictors of BMI among adults with Down syndrome: the social context of health promotion. *Res. Devel. Disability.*, 1997 18, 261–274.

Harris N, Rosenberg A, Jangda S. Prevalence of obesity in International Special Olympic athletes as determined by body mass index. *J. Am. Diet Assoc.,* 2003 103, 235-237

Luke, A; Roizen, NJ; Sutton, M; Schoeller, DA. Energy expenditure in children with Down syndrome: correcting metabolic rate for movement. *J. Pediatr.,* 1994 125, 829–838.

McDermott S, Platt T, Krishnaswami S. Are individuals with mental retardation living in the community at high risk for chronic disease? *Family Medicine* 1997, 20, 429-34.

Melville, CA; Cooper, SA; McGrother, CW; Thorp, CF; Collacott, R. Obesity in adults with Down syndrome: a case-control study. *J. Intellec. Disabilit. Research,* 2005 49, 125-133.

Moran, R; Drane, W; McDermott, S; Dasari, S; Scurry, JB; Platt, T. Obesity among people with and without Mental Retardation across adulthood. *Obes. Res.,* 2005 13, 342-349.

National Institute of Diabetes and Digestive and Kidney Disease, Weight- control Information Network. Obesity, Physical Activity and Weight Control Glossary. 2007 July 30. Available from: http://win.niddk.nih,gov/publications/glossary.htm#index.

Prasher VP. Overweight and obesity amongst Down's syndrome adults. *J. Intellect. Disabil. Res.,* 1995 16, 489-499.

Rimmer, JH; Braddock, D; Fujiura, G. Prevalence of obesity in adults with MR: implications for health promotion and disease prevention. *Ment. Retard.,* 1993 31, 105-110.

Rimmer, JH; Wang, E. Obesity prevalence among a group of Chicago residents with disabilities. *Arch. Phys. Med. Rehabil.,* 2005 86, 1461-1464.

Rubin, SS; Rimmer, JH; Chicoine, B; Braddock, D; McGuire, DE. Overweight prevalence in persons with Down syndrome. *Ment. Retard.,* 1998 36, 175–181.

U.S. Department of Health and Human Services. *The surgeon general's call to action to prevent and decrease overweight and obesity.* Washington, DC: U.S. Government Printing Office; 2001.

Yamaki, K. Body weight status among adults with intellectual disability in the community. *Ment. Retard.,* 2005 43, 1-10.

Chapter IV

Hypertension

The Research Questions: What is the prevalence of hypertension among adults with developmental disabilities and how does this compare to other adults, after controlling for established risk factors? For those adults who do not have hypertension when they enter the family medicine practice sites under study, are there differences in the incidence of hypertension among the impairment groups compared to those without a disability?

Definition of Hypertension and Prevalence in the General Population: Hypertension is defined as high blood pressure, a measurement of higher than desired force applied to the walls of the arteries as the heart pumps blood through the body. Blood pressure is influenced by the force and amount of blood pumped, and the size and flexibility of the arteries. Blood pressure is continually changing depending on activity, temperature, diet, emotional state, posture, physical health, and medication use. The evidence based standard for diagnosing hypertension has changed a number of times during the past two decades however hypertension generally means the systolic blood pressure is consistently over 140 or the diastolic blood pressure is consistently over 90. The Seventh Report of the Joint National Committee on Prevention, Detection, Evaluation, and Treatment of High Blood Pressure added a category for "prehypertension" defined as blood pressure 120/80 mmHg to 139/89 mmHg (Chobanian et al, 2003). The prehypertensive level was not included in our study.

The prevalence of hypertension was reported in the third National Health and Nutrition Examination Survey (NHANES) as 28.4 percent for adults over 18 years of age and the prevalence of hypertension increases sharply with advancing age. The age-adjusted prevalence in the non-Hispanic black and non-Hispanic white populations was 32.4% and 23.3% respectively. Overall, two thirds of the people with hypertension were aware of their diagnosis (69%), and a majority took prescribed medications (53%) (Burt, Whelton, Roccella et al, 1995; Fields, Burt, Cutler et al, 2004). Age is a well established risk factor for hypertension, with prevalence as high as 60% for adults over the age of 65 years. Gender is not a risk factor and in recent reports isolated systolic hypertension was present in two thirds of the older men and women who had hypertension (Aronow et al, 2006). Hypertension is not a disease state; it is an important risk factor for the morbidity and mortality associated with cardiovascular disease (CVD) and cerebrovascular accidents (CVA or stroke).

Literature Review of Hypertension in Adults with Developmental Disability: Some recent reports indicate that cardiovascular disease related deaths are greater for persons with mental retardation than for the general population (Hill, Gridley, Cnattingius et al, 2003; Day, Strauss, Shavelle et al, 2005). These finding needs to be assessed in terms of the specific circumstances of people with developmental disabilities, such as where they reside, and how much support they receive. Adults with MR who reside in community settings among their peers without disabilities, have a CVD prevalence of 42% compared to 32% for the adults who still live in institutions. Likewise, those with mild to moderate MR have higher prevalence (55%) of CVD compared to those with severe/profound MR (26%) (Janicki and MacEachron et al, 1984; Janicki and Jacobson et al, 1986).

The prevalence of both cardiovascular disease and hypertension varies by the type of setting in which individuals live and by the country in which they reside. International studies have reported lower prevalence of CVD and hypertensive diseases among adults with cognitive disabilities (Draheim, 2006; van den Akker, Maaskant, and van der Meijden et al, 2006). The range of reported prevalence of hypertension among studies conducted in the US is from 10-23% for those with severe MR to 25-41% for those with mild to moderate MR (Draheim, 2006; McDermott, Platt, and Krishnaswami et al, 1997; Kapell, Nightingale, Rodriguez, Lee and Zigman et al, 1998; Draheim et al, 2002, McCubbin, Williams et al, 2002). When comparisons are made about risk factors independent of disease processes the results are somewhat different. Frequencies of age-related cardiovascular risk factors, including hypertension and hyperlipidemia were compared for adults with developmental disabilities to data from the National Health and Nutrition Evaluation Survey III and it was found that adults with developmental disability had a lower overall reported frequency of these risk factors (Janicki, Davidson, Henderson, McCallion, Taets, Force, Sulkes, Frangenber, and Ladrigan et al, 2002).

People with Down syndrome have a substantially different profile for cardiovascular disease compared to others with mental retardation. It is well established that congenital heart defects (CHD) are associated with Down syndrome, and the prevalence of CHD has been reported as high as 50% in young children with Down syndrome (Geggel, O'Brien, Feingold, 1993; Goldhaber, Brown, Sutton et al, 1987). However, studies have shown that while individuals with Down syndrome are more likely to be obese and have high cholesterol profiles, they typically have low blood pressure (Rimmer, Braddock, and Marks et al, 1995; Draheim, McCubbin, and Williams et al, 2002a) and low prevalence of non-congenital cardiovascular disease (Yla-Herttuala, Luoma, Nikkari, Kivimaki et al, 1989). Despite evidence that adults with Down syndrome have lower than typical blood pressure, in a comprehensive review article on care of adults with Down syndrome typical screening for hypertension is recommended (Smith et al, 2001).

What is the Conceptual Framework for this question?: Cardiovascular disease is a broad term that includes hypertension, coronary heart disease, and cerebral vascular disease. There have been numerous risk factors identified for CVD including hypertension, sedentary activity levels, smoking, increased low-density lipoprotein (LDL), decreased high-density lipoprotein (HDL), obesity, diabetes, and family history of CVD. The oldest routinely used and relatively objective measure of CVD risk is blood pressure monitoring at physician visits.

The literature is clear that cardiovascular disease develops as a result of genetic predisposition, lifestyle behaviors, and the aging process. These factors are difficult to assess, challenging to alter, and complex in their interaction, thus individual risk assessment is only possible to a limited degree. For most adults with mental retardation with no known genetic cause of their MR, the range of genetic predisposition for heart disease and survival expectations are likely as varied as it is for the general population. For some adults with mental retardation associated with a genetic syndrome, such as Down syndrome, the incidence and prevalence of cardiovascular disease has been studied and for others it is unknown.

An important difference in adults with developmental disabilities compared to the general population is the higher likelihood that adults with DD are unemployed and more likely to be poor. However, it is not clear whether adults with developmental disabilities are more or less active and whether they eat a healthy diet compared to the general population.

There is some evidence in the literature that the prevalence of cardiovascular disease (CVD) in adults with mental retardation is greater and the onset is earlier than in the general population (Janicki and Jacobson et al, 1986; Rimmer, Braddock, and Marks et al, 1995; Draheim, McCubbin, and Williams et al, 2006). However, the CVD experience for adults with Down syndrome in adulthood appears to be similar to the experience of the general population and age-appropriate screening for cardiovascular risk factors is recommended (Smith et al, 2001). And the CVD experience of adults with cerebral palsy, autism and MR with psychiatric disability is not described in the literature.

For individuals who make regular office visits a surveillance system is in place in nearly every clinic and office to alert the physician about hypertension. Measurement of blood pressure using a sphygmotonometer is routine in almost all clinical environments. Hypertension is a preventable and treatable condition that is reversible for some individuals who modify their diet and physical activity. A number of modifiable factors have been implicated in the development of hypertension, including salt intake, obesity, occupation, alcohol intake, family size, stimulant intake, excessive noise exposure and crowding (van Kempen, Kruize, and Boshuizen et al, 2002; van den Akker, Maaskant, and van der Meijden et al, 2006). A few of these factors are thought to be highly prevalent in the lives of adults with developmental disabilities, most notably inadequate physical activity and unemployment (Draheim, 2006). The extent to which excessive noise is present in large group homes or sheltered workshops is variable and the concern about crowding is probably limited to residents of large group facilities and some large family settings. Because hypertension is amenable to treatment it is important to compare the onset and course of management for people with developmental disabilities compared to a comparison group.

Given the potential for prevention and treatment of high blood pressure the focus of this chapter is on the incidence and prevalence of hypertension. We will also present data on the prevalence of coronary artery disease since this is also a well documented condition in family medicine physician medical records.

Case Study: CJ is a 55 year old male with cerebral palsy (ICD 9 343.2), seizure disorder (780.39), hypertension (401.9) and mild mental retardation (ICD0 317) who moved to an ICF – MR in 1990 from his family home where he was cared for by his aging mother. At the time of his admission he used a wheelchair and was 66 inches tall and weighed 255 pounds (BMI 41). CJ became of a patient of Dr. F, a family medicine physician practicing in the same town as the ICF. Dr. F. noted that CJ had severe edema of his lower extremities and blood pressure that fluctuated from 135/90-160/110. Dr. F. also noted in his clinical record that CJ was a non-smoker. When Dr. F. started caring for CJ his hypertension was very poorly controlled and he was on 3 medications. Through medication adjustments and dietary restriction, his weight gradually decreased over the next 5 years to 180 pounds which reduced his BMI to 29. Some range of motion exercises for his contracted lower limbs also minimally reduced the edema. At that time his blood pressure was controlled with 20 mg of lisinopril (Prinivil).

Four years ago, because CJ had many adaptive skills he was moved to a community training home (CTH – II), a less restrictive environment, which was determined to be a more appropriate setting for him. He continued to be a patient of Dr. F. since they had established a positive doctor patient relationship, despite a somewhat longer drive to the medical practice site. In the course of the next 4 years, because CJ had a more unrestricted diet and a sedentary lifestyle he gained back a large percentage of the weight he had lost.

Dr. F referred CJ to a nutrition counselor and CJ attended a community based education program about the importance of healthy diet and physical activity. Six months after completing the education program CJ had increased to 220 pounds and his BMI was up to 36. Dr. F. added hydrochlorothiazide (Microzide) and amlodipine besylate/atorvastatin calcium (Caduet) to his hypertensive regime and his blood pressure was usually 135/85. CJ continues to receive education to help to make better food choices and he is now requesting to be moved to a supervised apartment setting.

Our Research Findings: The standards for diagnosing hypertension changed during and after our study period of 1990-2003 thus we used the evidence based standard that applied at the time the diagnosis was made. Table 1 shows the prevalence of hypertension among the adults with developmental disabilities was 28%. For the comparison group the prevalence of hypertension was 42%. Thus, without consideration of risk factor status, it appears the risk was higher for the comparison group for ever having hypertension at some time during the seven or more years people were receiving care at the two sites.

We have data on a number of the well established risk factors for the development of hypertension. These risks include race, age, body mass index (BMI), diabetes, and smoking. When we tested these factors using logistic regression modeling with the study subjects it is noteworthy that all of the potential confounders have a level at which there was significantly elevated risks for hypertension. Patients who are African-American had an odds ratio of 1.91 compared to the whites ($p<0.001$), for each year of age the odds ratio was 1.06 ($p<0.001$), for each increase in BMI the odds ratio was 1.09 ($p<0.001$), diabetes was associated with an increased odds ratio of 3.09 ($p<0.001$) and smoking was associated with an increased odds ratio of 1.56 ($p<0.001$).

The odds ratios for hypertension, after controlling for these confounders, for each of the DD groups are shown in Table 2. When all of the confounders were in the predictive logistic regression models the adjusted odds ratio (and 95% confidence interval) was not statistically significantly different for any of the developmental disability groups compared to the comparison group. Thus, the differences in risk factors, not the disability status of the individuals was accounting for the prevalence rates shown in Table 1.

We also explored the onset of new cases of hypertension during the period patients in the study were receiving care at the two sites. In this analysis we excluded all those with hypertension already established in their medical record and looked at only those individuals who had normal blood pressure when they entered care. In this case we used survival analysis to do the modeling (Table 3). Again, we tested the well established risk factors for their contribution to the development of hypertension. These risks were race, gender, body mass index (BMI), diabetes, and smoking. And again these factors have a level at which there was significantly elevated risk for developing hypertension. Patients who are African-American had a hazard ratio of 1.82 compared to the whites ($p<0.001$), for each increase in BMI the hazard ratio was 1.06 ($p<0.001$), and females a protective effect with a hazard ratio of 0.86 ($p<0.043$). Then when these risk factors were in the survival analysis, using Cox proportional hazard modeling, along with disability status, there was no difference in the risk for developing hypertension between the adults with and without developmental disabilities.

Implications for Case Study: The dynamic and complex factors involved in CJ's life are impacting his ability to control his hypertension. His family physician needs to understand the context in which CJ is living in order to alter his medical management and maintain a hopeful outlook about his disease. At any point in his adult life a snapshot of CJ's life could reflect very different disease states and prognoses. Thus, it is important for his physician to understand the levels of care and support being offered in order to manage his treatment. Hypertension is not a static disease and as CJ moved through different levels of independent living the challenges in terms of diet, physical activity, stress and the impact on his weight and cardiovascular fitness level changed. At the age of 55 years CJ still has the opportunity to achieve better control of his weight and hypertension. A family physician monitors CJ's blood pressure on a regular basis (approximately 4 times a year), checks on his compliance with all of his medications, makes changes in CJ's medication when needed, and orders diagnostic tests to identify changes in risk factors or disease progression on a regular basis.

Table 1. Prevalence of hypertension among adults without disability and those with developmental disability, by sub-group and risk factors

Prevalence (ever)	Without disability	All DD	Autism	Down syndrome	Cerebral Palsy	MR with Psychiatric Illness	MR
Number	1809	694	54	58	163	152	267
Prevalence for Group	41.6	28.2	14.8	17.2	22.1	36.2	32.6
Gender							
Male	38.8	28.2	19.1	14.7	25.7	31.1	33.8
Female	43.7	28.3	0.0	20.8	19.1	41.0	31.2
Race							
White	34.6	25.8	13.2	16.3	18.9	28.0	35.3
African American	49.5	32.4	20.0	21.4	28.6	44.2	29.1
Other	21.9	0.0	0.0	0.0	0.0	0.0	0.0
Severity of primary condition							
Mild	n/a	n/a	10.0	33.3	32.0	43.3	45.9
Moderate	n/a	n/a	18.0	12.5	16.1	19.1	25.0
Severe	n/a	n/a	0.0	15.9	19.3	29.3	24.8
Residential Type							
Least Restrictive Environment	n/a	34.8	33.3	25.0	30.0	34.8	38.9
Most Restrictive Environment	n/a	20.4	12.5	18.8	20.7	27.8	18.8

Table 2. Adjusted* Odds Ratio for each developmental disability group

Group	n	Prevalence	Adjusted* Odds Ratio	Lower Confidence Interval	Upper Confidence Interval	P-Value
Comparison	1809	41.6	1.00			
Autism	54	14.8	0.91	0.17	4.76	0.910
Cerebral Palsy	163	17.2	1.04	0.27	4.03	0.950
Down syndrome	58	22.1	0.59	0.12	3.01	0.523
MR with Psychiatric Illness	152	36.2	0.75	0.17	3.32	0.700
MR Only	267	32.6	0.81	0.19	3.48	0.772

*adjusted for practice site, age, race, gender, tobacco use, diabetes and starting BMI.

Table 3. Hazard Ratio* for development of hypertension for each developmental disability group

Groups	n	Hazard Ratio	P-Value
Comparisons	1635		
Autism	53	1.40	0.352
Cerebral Palsy	159	1.06	0.746
Down syndrome	57	0.65	0.177
MR with Psychiatric Illness	145	0.90	0.463
MR Only	253	0.83	0.124

*adjusted for practice site, race, gender, tobacco use, diabetes and starting BMI.

Implications from our study findings: Our study suggests that people with developmental disabilities have comparable incidence and prevalence rates of hypertension as the comparison group from the same community. Our multiple variable analyses findings are interesting since none of the results indicate a statistically significant difference in the overall odds of developing hypertension, after controlling for risk factors and there is no difference in the risk for developing hypertension for those adults who enter the family medicine study sites without hypertension.

The overall prevalence of hypertension is high, approximately 30-40% of adults with and without developmental disabilities in our study. Thus, since hypertension is a known risk factor for cardiovascular disease it is clear that research should focus on identifying efficacious health promotion programs and strategies for all adults that will reduce hypertension while promoting physical activity and healthy eating.

References

Aronow WS. Heart disease and aging. *Med. Clin. N. Am.,* 2006 90, 849-862.

Chobanian AV. The seventh report of the Joint National Committee on Prevention, Detection, Evaluation, and Treatment of High Blodo Pressure: the JNC 7 report. *JAMA,* 2003 289, 2560-2572.

Burt VL, Whelton P, Roccella EJ, Brown C, Cutler JA, Higgins M, Horan MJ, Labarthe D. Prevalence of hypertension in the U.S. adult population. Results from the National Health and Nutrition Examination Survey 1988-1991. *Hypertension,* 1995, 305-313.

Day SM, Strauss DJ, Shavelle RM, Reynolds RJ. Mortality and causes of death in persons with Down syndrome in California. *Dev. Med. Child Neurol.,* 2005 47, 171-176.

Draheim CC. Cardiovascular disease prevalence and risk factors of persons with mental retardation. *Mental Retardation and Developmental Disabilities Research Reviews* 2006, 12, 3-12.

Draheim CC, McCubbin JA, Williams DP. Differences in cardiovascular disease risk between nondiabetic adults with mental retardation with and without Down syndrome. *Am. J. Ment. Retard,* 2002 107, 201-11.

Fields LE, Burt VL, Cutler JA, Hughes J, Roccella EJ, Sorlie P. The burden of adult hypertension in the United States 1999 to 2000: a rising tide. *Hypertension*, 2004 44, 398-404.

Geggel RL, O'Brien JE, Feingold M. Development of valve dysfunction in adolescents and young adults with Down syndrome and no know congenital hart disease. *J. Pediatr.* 1993; 122, 821-3.

Goldhaber SZ, Brown WD, Sutton MG. High frequency of mitral valve prolapse and aortic regurgitation among asymptomatic adults with Down's syndrome. *JAMA*, 1987 258, 1793-1795.

Hill DA, Gridley G, Cnattingius S, et al. Mortality and Cancer Incidence Among Individuals With Down Syndrome. *Arch. Intern. Med.,* 2003 163, 705-711.

Janicki MP, Davidson PW, Henderson CM, McCallion P, et al. Health characteristics and health services utilization in older adults with intellectual disability living in community residences. *J. Intellect. Disabil. Res.,* 2002 46, 287-298.

Janicki MB, Jacobson JW. Generational trends in sensory, physical, and behavioral abilities among older mentally retarded persons. *Am. J. Ment. Defic.* 1986 90, 490-500.

Janicki MB, MacEachron AE. Residential, health, and social service needs of elderly developmentally disabled persons. *Gerontologist.* 1984; 24:128-37.

Kapell D, Nightingale B, Rodriguez A, Lee JH, Zigman, WB, Schupf N. Prevalence of chronic medical conditions in adults with mental retardation: comparison with the general population. *Men. Retard.,* 1998 36, 269-79.

McDermott, S., Platt, T, Krishnaswami, S. "Are individuals with mental retardation living in the community at high risk for chronic disease?" *Fam. Med.,* 1997 29, 429-434.

Rimmer JH, Braddock D, Marks B. Health characteristics and behaviors of adults with mental retardation residing in three living arrangements. *Res. Dev. Disabil.,* 1995 16, 489-499.

Smith, D. Health care management of adults with Down syndrome. *American Family Physician.* 2001 64, 1031-1038.

van den Akker M, Maaskant MA, van der Meijden RJ. Cardiac diseases in people with intellectual disability. *J. Intellect. Disabil. Res.,* 2006 50, 515-22.

van Kempen EMM, Kruize H, Boshuizen HC. The Association between Noise Exposure and Blood Pressure and Ischemic Heart Disease: A Meta-analysis. *Environmental Health Perspectives* 2002, 110, 307-17.

Yla-Herttuala S, Luoma J, Nikkari T, Kivimaki T. Down's syndrome and atherosclerosis. *Atherosclerosis.* 1989 76, 269-272.

Chapter V

Diabetes

The Research Questions: What is the prevalence of diabetes among adults with developmental disabilities and how does this compare to other adults, after controlling for known risk factors? For those adults who do not have diabetes when they enter the family medicine practice sites under study, are there differences in the incidence of diabetes among the impairment groups compared to those without a disability?

Definition of Diabetes and Prevalence in the General Population: Diabetes mellitus is defined as inappropriate glucose metabolism leading to impaired removal of glucose from the circulation. While insulin mediates the clearance of glucose from blood, absolute or relative lack of insulin and/or impaired insulin action at its receptor causes delayed metabolism of circulating glucose (Schwartz and Kahn et al, 1999; Clark, Jones, de Koning, Hansen, and Matthews et al, 2001; Butler, Janson, Bonner-Weir, Ritzel, Rizza, and Butler et al, 2003; Ashcroft and Rorsman et al, 2004). Type 1 diabetes is caused by autoimmune destruction of pancreatic b-cells and failure to make insulin with the usual onset in childhood. Type 2 diabetes, also known as non-insulin dependent diabetes mellitus, is the most prevalent form of diabetes and onset is often during adulthood. Type 2 diabetics have iinsulin resistance, so that insulin produced by the pancreas cannot get inside fat and muscle cells to produce energy. As a result of insufficient insulin in the cells the pancreas produces more insulin and hyperglycemia and high blood insulin levels co-exist in the same individual. People who are overweight have a higher risk of insulin resistance, because fat interferes with the body's ability to use insulin. In addition, ssedentary life-style and metabolic syndrome are well-established risk factors for onset of Type 2 diabetes (Ristow, 2004).

The overall incidence of diabetes mellitus in the general population is 4–8% (Zimmet, Alberti, and Shaw et al, 2001). The CDC reported the prevalence of diagnosed diabetes for the age group 45-64 was 8.57%, and for those ages 65-74 it was 15.43% for the year 2000 (CDC, 2007). During 2005 the total prevalence of diabetes in the United States, for all ages, was 7.0% of the population. African Americans had substantially higher rates compared to whites, with black females having prevalence of 13.3% for all non-Hispanic blacks aged 20 years and older. In South Carolina, where over 30% of the population is African American, the prevalence of diagnosed diabetes in 2002 was 12.7% for adults 45-64 years of age and

18.3% in those 65-74 years of age. (Centers for Disease Control and Prevention et al, 2005; South Carolina Department of Health and Environmental Control et al, 2003).

Literature Review of Diabetes in Adults with Developmental Disability: According to the criteria of the World Health Organization (WHO) type 1 diabetes mellitus predominantly affects younger individuals, women who are pregnant, and a group that includes various syndromes, including Down syndrome, Klinefelter's syndrome, Prader-Willi syndrome, and Turner's syndrome (Alberti and Zimmet et al, 1998). Some medical and nursing textbooks and articles state "Diabetes mellitus develops in at least 1% of children and adolescents with Down syndrome" (Rubin and Crocker, 2006). However, the evidence is from a Danish study that used on a population based health registry to establish the prevalence of type 1 diabetes among people with Down syndrome was 0.7% (95% CI 0.3-1.35%) compared to the general population prevalence of 0.17% (95% CI 0.16-0.18%). This is an odds ratio of 4.12 (95% CI 2.1-8.2) (Bergholdt, Eising, Nerup, and Pociot et al, 2006).

There is limited literature on Type 2 diabetes mellitus in people with developmental disabilities. When frequencies of age-related cardiovascular risk factors, including adult-onset diabetes were compared to data from the National Health and Nutrition Evaluation Survey III, adults with developmental disabilities had a lower prevalence rates. Adult-onset diabetes was reported about twice as frequently in the NHANES-III cohort as compared to the cohort of 1,371 adults with ID aged 40-79 years living in small group, community based residences in two representative areas of New York State (Janicki, Davidson, Henderson, McCallion, Taets, and Force et al, 2002).

We previously analyzed and published a report comparing 366 adults with MR, living in the community, to two comparison groups without MR. We found individuals with MR had lower rates of the combined Type 1 and 2 diabetes compared to Medicaid and insured patients without developmental delay (McDermott, Platt, and Krishnaswami et al, 1997). More recently we published an article on the prevalence of diabetes in adults with disabilities including developmental disabilities (McDermott, Moran, Platt, Wood, Isaac, Dasari, 2007).

What is the Conceptual Framework for this question?: The association of Down syndrome and Type 1 diabetes is accepted by most physicians but there is little evidence to substantiate the higher prevalence. And since only 8-10% of people diagnosed with MR have Down syndrome the question about prevalence of both Type 1 and Type 2 diabetes for the remaining group of people with developmental disabilities remains open. The reasons to expect a higher prevalence of Type 2 diabetes in people with DD is based on the risk factors for its development including obesity, sedentary lifestyle, and hyperlipidemia. It is well documented that positive lifestyle changes in people at risk for development of type 2 diabetes can reduce the risk significantly (Eriksson and Lindgarde et al, 1991; Tuomilehto, Lindstrom, and Eriksson et al, 2001). However, these changes are hard to make unless they are encouraged and supported in the home environment. Our observation has been that adults with developmental disabilities respond to the limitations imposed on them in most environments and the more restrictive the setting (large group homes represent the most restrictive community living, followed by supervised apartments, family living, and independent living) the less likely residents indulge in overeating and sedentary lifestyles.

Thus, we expect adults with DD who live in an unstructured or unsupervised arrangement are at increased risk for developing type 2 diabetes compared to adults with DD living in more restrictive environments.

Case Study: At the age 29 years, while living at an intermediate care facility (ICF-MR) KD developed insulin dependent diabetes (ICD9 250.00). KD received primary care from a family medicine physician, Dr. T. practicing in the University/ County Hospital based family medicine center. Dr. T. first met KD when she was 30 years old and she noted KD's condition is complicated by mental retardation that was at the moderate level (ICD9 318.0), seizure disorder (ICD9 780.39) and obsessive eating disorder, that made dietary control difficult. The ICF-MR staff transported KD to a workshop 5 days a week where there was often easy access to other client's and staff food. Attempts to control KD on oral medications, proved unsuccessful and Dr. T. transitioned her to 75/25 insulin lispro protamine and insulin lispro injection (Humalog), in addition to pioglitazone hydrochloride (Actos) that was titrated up to 75 mg once a day. Initially KD was administered her medication by the ICF-MR nurse but over the course of a year she learned to do it herself, under close supervision. KD's seizure disorder was controlled with divalproex sodium (Depakote) which seemed to improve her impulsive and obsessive behaviors.

By the time KD was 34 years old Dr. T. adjusted her insulin dose multiple times per year and she was even given a sliding scale for dosage to administer due to wide varying glucose readings. Once again staff assumed primary responsibility for the injections. The staff reported to Dr. T. that their greatest difficulty was in controlling the late afternoon and evening glucose level due to KD's erratic dietary intake and her access to restricted foods. She continued to gain weight over subsequent years and actually gained 35 pounds from the time of her diagnosis. KD is now 38 years old and Dr. T. monitors her for the development of complications of diabetes. At this stage KD has not developed any of the complications of diabetes, but her hemoglobin A1C has ranged from 7.0 to over to 11 but is usually in the 8-9 range.

Our Research Findings: Diabetes Mellitus was identified in both progress notes and problem lists combined with notations about and actual clinical laboratory results. The diagnosis of diabetes has been modified on numerous occasions in the past 20 years so we used the evidence based definition that applied at the time the diagnosis was made in the clinical record. Diabetes severity was based on laboratory values, medications and physician notations. Severity of diabetes is also subject to change over time, and in this case an individual can move from more to less severe or visa versa. Cases were considered mild if the glucose level was <200 and/or the HgA1C was less than 7 and the physician prescribed a lifestyle modification program with increases in exercise and diet restrictions and/or oral drugs were prescribed. Moderate diabetes was coded if the glucose level was between 200-300, HgA1C was 7.0-9.0 and insulin was prescribed, with or without other oral medications. Severe diabetes was "brittle" or "uncontrolled" with other systems involvement, glucose >300, and HgA1C greater than 9.0.

Table 1. Prevalence of diabetes among adults without disability and those with developmental disability, by sub-group and risk factors

Prevalence (ever)	Patients without disability	All DD	Autism	Down Syndrome	Cerebral Palsy	MR with Psychiatric Illness	MR
All	1809	694	54	58	163	152	267
	15.2	9.9	1.8	8.6	6.1	11.8	13.1
Gender							
Male	13.9	9.2	2.4	8.8	4.1	10.8	13.1
Female	16.1	10.8	0.0	8.3	7.9	12.8	13.1
Race							
White	10.1	8.9	0.0	4.7	7.6	9.3	13.1
African American	20.0	11.8	6.7	21.4	3.6	14.3	13.6
Other	17.1	0.0	0.0	0.0	0.0	0.0	0.0
Severity of Primary Disability							
Mild	n/a	n/a	0.0	16.7	12.0	14.4	16.3
Moderate	n/a	n/a	2.6	0.0	5.4	14.3	16.7
Severe	n/a	n/a	0.0	9.1	1.8	4.9	8.3
Residential Type							
Least Restrictive Environment	n/a	7.1	0.0	8.3	0.0	4.4	11.1
Most Restrictive Environment	n/a	4.9	0.0	6.3	1.7	2.8	8.8

When we looked at the prevalence of diabetes in the patients without disability and those with developmental disabilities we observed the prevalence was highest for the comparison patients and lowest for those with autism (Table 1).

In general, women had higher prevalence of diabetes compared to men and African Americans had higher prevalence compared to whites. It is also noteworthy that those with milder forms of developmental disabilities and those living in less restrictive environments had higher prevalence of diabetes compared to their counterparts with more severe disabilities and more restrictive living environments.

We explored the prevalence of diabetes by decade of life, shown in Table 2. It appears increasing age is somewhat associated with diabetes.

Table 2. Prevalence of diabetes, by disability and age group

	Age in Decades				
Group	20 - 29	30-40	40-50	50-60	60+
Comparison	18.9	26.7	23.9	24.8	23.9
All DD	17.6	18.3	13.6	18.5	9.1
Autism	5.0	-	-	-	-
Down syndrome	10.7	7.7	22.2	12.5	-
Cerebral Palsy	15.9	15.8	10.7	10.0	.0
MR with psychiatric Illness	30.9	23.7	29.0	23.5	9.1
MR Only	18.6	20.6	5.8	21.4	5.9

We used logistic regression modeling to explore the risk for diabetes among those with developmental disabilities compared to controls without disability after controlling for age, race, gender, BMI, and tobacco use. The risk factors that were statistically significant in their association with diabetes were race (Adjusted Odds Ratio 2.17: 95% Confidence Interval 1.65-2.86, $p<0.001$), age (for each year Adjusted Odds Ratio 1.05: 95% Confidence Interval 1.04-1.07, $p<0.001$), and BMI when they entered the practice (for each BMI increase Adjusted Odds Ratio 1.09: 95% Confidence Interval 1.07-1.11, $p<0.001$). After controlling for these risk factors there were no statistically significant differences in the odds of having diabetes for adults with developmental disabilities compared to those without disabilities in the same practice (Table 3).

Table 3. Logistic Regression, adjusted* odds ratio for prevalence of diabetes, by group

Groups	n	Prevalence	Adjusted Odds Ratio	Lower Confidence Interval	Upper Confidence Interval	P-Value
Comparison	1809	15.2	1.00			
Autism	54	1.8	0.33	0.04	2.56	0.289
Cerebral Palsy	163	8.6	1.12	0.56	2.24	0.750
Down syndrome	58	6.1	1.10	0.41	2.95	0.849
MR with Psychiatric Illness	152	11.8	1.06	0.60	1.85	0.845
MR Only	267	13.1	1.32	0.86	2.02	0.208

* adjusted for medical site, age, race, gender, BMI, tobacco use.

We also explored the onset of diabetes among the adults who entered the practice without diabetes using survival analysis. Three known risk factors were statistically significant in their association with diabetes. African Americans had a hazard rate of 2.09 ($p<0.001$), and for each increase of BMI at which an individual started care at the two sites the hazard rate was 1.07 ($p<0.001$). Table 4 shows that after controlling for these risk factors, using Cox proportional hazard modeling there was no group with developmental disabilities where the risk for developing diabetes was statistically significantly different from the comparison group.

Table 4. Survival Analysis Hazard Rate* for developing diabetes, by group

Groups	N	Hazard Ratio	P-Value
Comparison	1733		
Autism	54	0.54	0.545
Cerebral Palsy	161	0.85	0.618
Down syndrome	57	1.09	0.851
MR with Psychiatric Illness	152	0.90	0.680
MR Only	258	1.03	0.860

*adjusting for medical site, race, gender, tobacco use and starting BMI.

We conducted analysis to compare the onset of diabetes among adults with obesity since it is well established that obesity is a risk factor for the development of adult onset diabetes. It should be noted that in our study people with developmental disabilities were less likely to be obese, compared to controls. Table 5 shows the percent of adults with diabetes among adults who were obese. Column two has the adults without disability and columns 3-8 shows the percent for those with developmental disabilities.

Table 5. Percent with diabetes among adults *with obesity*, by disability subgroup

	Patients without disability	All DD	Autism	Down syndrome	Cerebral Palsy	MR with Psychiatric Illness	MR Only
Number	834	276	22	36	34	70	114
Percent	23.3	17.4	4.6	13.9	20.6	15.7	21.1
Gender							
Male	23.8	17.1	5.9	15.8	8.3	23.1	20.0
Female	23.0	17.7	0.0	11.8	27.3	11.4	22.0
Race							
White	17.2	15.2	0.0	7.1	21.7	12.1	21.5
African American	27.0	20.9	16.7	37.5	18.2	18.9	20.8
Other	33.3	-	-	-	-	-	-

Table 6. Adjusted* Odds Ratio using Logistic regression for diabetes for only those with obesity

Groups	n	Prevalence	Adjusted* Odds Ratio	Lower Confidence Interval	Upper Confidence Interval	P-Value
Comparison	834	23.2	1.00			
Autism	22	4.6	0.46	0.06	3.51	0.449
Cerebral Palsy	34	20.6	1.56	0.64	3.79	0.327
Down syndrome	36	13.9	0.98	0.36	2.70	0.970
MR with Psychiatric Illness	70	15.7	0.81	0.40	1.63	0.554
MR Only	114	21.1	1.25	0.75	2.09	0.400

* adjusted for medical site, age, race, gender, BMI, tobacco use.

We used logistic regression modeling to explore the association of known risk factors among adults with pre-existing obesity, for diabetes. Being African-American was associated with a statistically significant risk for diabetes (Adjusted Odds Ratio 2.11, 95% Confidence Interval 1.53-2.93, p<0.001). Each year of age also had a statistically significant risk (Adjusted Odds Ratio 1.06, 95% Confidence Interval 1.05-1.07, p<0.001). Table 6 shows the odds ratio for diabetes, among those with pre-existing obesity, after controlling for these known risk factors. None of the sub-groups with developmental disabilities had statistically significant different odds for diabetes compared to those without disability, when only those with prior obesity were included in the logistic regression models, after controlling for race and age.

Finally, we explored the onset of diabetes among those patients who did not have diabetes when they entered the practices although they did have established obesity. Again, when we controlled for risk factors, there was no difference in the risk for onset of diabetes for any of the sub-groups with developmental disabilities compared to those without disabilities (Table 7).

Table 7. Adjusted* Hazard Ratio using Cox Proportional Hazard Modeling for developing diabetes when patients had pre-existing obesity

Groups	n	Adjusted* Hazard Ratio	P-Value
Comparison	834		
Autism	22	0.69	0.713
Cerebral Palsy	34	1.25	0.573
Down syndrome	36	0.96	0.937
MR with Psychiatric Illness	70	0.75	0.355
MR Only	114	1.04	0.869

* adjusted for medical site, age, race, gender, BMI, tobacco use.

Implications from our study findings: Our study findings show no difference in the prevalence or incidence of diabetes among adults with and without developmental disabilities, even though the crude rates appear to be substantially higher among those without disabilities and those in the two groups with mental retardation. These crude rates are highly influenced by the differences in the distribution of risk factors among the groups. In other words, people with developmental disabilities had lower crude rates of diabetes because the proportion of women and African-Americans was lower than in the comparison group. When we controlled for the risk factors there were no differences in the risk for diabetes in the groups. Even more importantly there was no difference in the groups with developmental disabilities compared to those without disabilities for odds of having diabetes or onset of diabetes among adults with established obesity.

Implications for Case Study: KD developed diabetes at age 29 years and she has struggled to modify her diet. Lifestyle modification is a challenge for all diabetics and the addition of KD's mental retardation, epilepsy, and mental health problems makes diet modification difficult. It is important for KD to have a continuing relationship with her family medicine physician, so that despite the challenges she faces, she will receive regular monitoring. It is clear that KD is at high risk for complications of diabetes including ulcerations, neuropathy, vision complications, and kidney failure and heart disease. Her physician needs to be alert to changes in her condition and order diagnostic tests, adjust her medications, and continue to encourage responsible self management behavior so complications can be minimized.

References

Alberti KGM.M, Zimmet PZ. Definition, diagnosis and classification of diabetes mellitus and its complications. I. diagnosis and classification of diabetes mellitus. Provisional report of a WHO Consultation. *Diabet Med.,* 1998 15, 539-553.

Ashcroft F, Rorsman P. Type 2 diabetes mellitus: not quite exciting enough? *Hum. Mol. Genet.,* 2004 13, 21–31.

Bergholdt R, Eising S, Nerup J, Pociot F. Increased prevalence of Down's syndrome in individuals with type 1 diabetes in Denmark: a nationwide population-based study. *Diabetologia,* 2006 49, 1179-82.

Butler AE, Janson J, Bonner-Weir S, Ritzel R, Rizza RA, Butler PC. Beta-cell deficit and increased beta-cell apoptosis in humans with type 2 diabetes. *Diabetes,* 2003 52,102–110.

Centers for Disease Control and Prevention. Prevalence of Diagnosed Diabetes per 100 Population, by Age, United Sates, 1980-2005. 2005. 2007 March 2. Available from:http://www.cdc.gov/diabetes/statistics/prev/national/tprevage.htm:

Clark A, Jones LC, de Koning E, Hansen BC, Matthews DR. Decreased insulin secretion in type 2 diabetes: a problem of cellular mass or function? *Diabetes,* 2001 50, S169–S171.

Eriksson KF, Lindgarde F. Prevention of type 2 (non-insulin-dependent) diabetes mellitus by diet and physical exercise. The 6-year Malmö feasibility study. *Diabetologia,* 1991 34, 891-8.

Janicki MP, Davidson PW, Henderson CM, McCallion P, Taets JD, Force LT, et al. Health characteristics and health services utilization in older adults with intellectual disability living in community residences. *J. Intellect. Disabil. Res.,* 2002 46, 287-298.

McDermott S, Moran R, Platt T, Wood H, Isaac T, Dasari S. Prevalence of diabetes in persons with disabilities. *Journal of Developmental and Physical Disabilities,* 2007, 19, 263-271.

McDermott S, Platt T, Krishnaswami S. Are individuals with mental retardation at high risk for chronic disease? *Fam. Med.,* 1997 29, 429-34.

Ristow M. Neurodegenerative disorders associated with diabetes mellitus. *J. Mol. Med.,* 2004 82, 510-529.

Rubin, IL and Crocker AC. *Medical care for children and adults with developmental disabilities.* 2006, Paul Brookes Publishing Co. Baltimore MD, 389.

South Carolina Department of Health and Environmental Control. *Burden of Diabetes Report* 2003, 25-38.

Schwartz MW, Kahn SE. Insulin resistance and obesity. *Nature,* 1999 402,860–861

Tuomilehto J, Lindstrom J, Eriksson JG, et al. Prevention of Type 2 Diabetes Mellitus by Changes in Lifestyle among Subjects with Impaired Glucose Tolerance. *N. Engl. J. Med.*, 2001 344, 1343-1350.

Zimmet P, Alberti KG, Shaw J. Global and societal implications of the diabetes epidemic. *Nature,* 2001 414, 782–787.

Chapter VI

Congestive Heart Failure

The Research Questions: What is the prevalence of congestive heart failure among adults with developmental disabilities and how does this compare to other adults, after controlling for known risk factors? For those adults who do not have congestive heart failure when they enter the family medicine practice sites under study, are there differences in the incidence of CHF between the impairment groups compared to those without a disability?

Definition of Congestive Heart Failure and Prevalence in the General Population: Congestive heart failure (CHF), or heart failure, is a condition in which the heart can't pump enough blood to the body's other organs. This can result from:

- narrowed arteries to the heart muscle — coronary artery disease
- myocardial infarction, with scar tissue
- high blood pressure
- heart valve disease due to past rheumatic fever or other causes
- cardiomyopathy
- congenital heart defects.
- endocarditis and/or myocarditis -infection of the heart valves and/or heart muscle (Aronow, Ahn, and Kronzon et al, 1998).

The symptoms of CHF include shortness of breath and tiredness. In addition, as blood flow out of the heart slows the blood returning through the veins backs up, causing congestion in the tissues and edema in the legs and ankles. In some people fluid collects in the lungs and interferes with breathing, causing shortness of breath, especially when a person is lying down. Heart failure also affects the kidneys' ability to dispose of sodium and water and increases the edema. Cardiomyopathy is primary disease of the heart muscle itself that is often caused by diabetes mellitus, hypertension, and alcohol abuse, as well as unknown causes. Thus, there are complex relationships between the chronic conditions that share common etiology and can result in comorbidity in the same individuals.

The prevalence and incidence of CHF increase with age and is the most common cause of hospitalization in persons aged 65 years and older (Kannel and Belanger et al, 1991; Aronow, Ahn, and Gutstein et al, 2002). The prevalence of CHF is approximately 2 percent for adults 40-59 years, 5 percent for those 60-69 years and over 10 percent for those over 70 years. The prevalence is approximately 25 percent higher among African-Americans compared to whites. There is no gender difference in prevalence or incidence. In the U.S. the incidence rate is approximately one in 679 people or 10 per 1,000 after the age of 65 years (NHLBI et al, 1996; Collins et al, 2002). The risk for onset is double in those with hypertension and five times greater in those who have had a myocardial infarction (NHLBI et al, 1996). The leading causes of heart failure are coronary artery disease, high blood pressure, and diabetes (NHLBI et al, 2007).

Literature Review of Congestive Heart Failure in Adults with Developmental Disability: Cardiac disease is a significant health problem and a main cause of death in people with developmental disabilities (van den Akker, Maaskant, and van der Maijden et al, 2006; Hayden et al, 1998; Patja, Molsa, and Iivanainen et al, 2001). We previously published an article about heart disease in adults with primary psychiatric illness, from this study (McDermott, Moran, Platt, Wood, Isaac, Dasari, 2005). However, there is no literature on the specific diagnosis of congestive heart failure in adults with DD.

What is the Conceptual Framework for this question?: The life expectancy of people with developmental disabilities is approaching their age matched peers and cardiovascular disease is the number one cause of death for both groups. Adults with developmental disabilities are exposed to difficult lifestyle choices as less restrictive residential alternatives become widespread. Clearly adults with developmental disabilities have some of the same lifestyle challenges as the general population, including physical inactivity, high fat diet, tobacco use, and obesity. Age-related changes in the cardiovascular system, overt and occult cardiovascular disease, and limited physical activity affect cardiovascular function in elderly persons (Aronow et al, 2006). Thus, the incidence and prevalence of congestive heart failure among adults with DD needs to be studied.

Case Study: Dr. A. has been the primary care physician for GM, a 59 year old male with mild mental retardation (ICD9 317) who received mitral valve replacement over 20 years ago. Throughout the years Dr. A. has collaborated with GM's cardiologist and cardiac surgeon. GM sees his specialist approximately once each year unless Dr. A. feels a consultation is needed. GM has chronic atrial fibrillation (ICD9 427.31) and received warfarin and anticoagulant coudmadin therapy. In addition, Dr. A. treats GM for hypercholesterolemia (ICD9 272.0) with atorvastatin calcium (Lipitor) and he manages his epilepsy (ICD9 780.39) with valporic acid (Depakene) and carbamazepine (Carbatrol). Annually GM also has a consultation appointment with a neurologist who writes a thorough note to Dr. A. about GM's epilepsy status and his prescribed medications.

Starting about 10 years ago during an annual consult with the cardiologist it was discovered that GM had mild cardiomyopathy with a decreased ejection fraction of about 40%. GM was on digoxin (Lanoxin), and during his cardiology consult furosemide was added to his regimen.

GM was stable and functional during this time while living in a supervised apartment. Due to his medication regime and his tendency to fatigue easily GM was unable to find work in the community, although this was his desire. Due to his valve replacement he was also receiving monthly penicillin G benzathine (bicillin). His multiple conditions required frequent visits to his family medicine physician who coordinates all of his care.

Starting about 6 months ago GM began to slowly lose weight and his ejection fraction dropped to 25%. No cause for his weight loss could be determined although he had an extensive workup. GM was becoming increasingly short of breath and he had some peripheral edema. Adjustments were made to his medication regimen and he was able to continue to live in the same supervised apartment. Although it was felt that his condition had finally stabilized, he died suddenly two months ago from what was thought to be either an acute myocardial infarction or acute pulmonary edema. He was scheduled to be admitted to the hospital for a workup but died on the day of his planned admission.

Our Research Findings: We first explored the prevalence of Congestive Heart Failure among adults without disability and with developmental disabilities. The crude prevalence rate was the highest among those without disabilities at 4.1 percent. There was no CHF among patients with autism and the range for the other developmental disability sub-groups was from a low of 1.7% for those with Down syndrome to a high of 3.3% for those with MR and psychiatric illness.

Since it is well established that risk for congestive heart failure is related to age, obesity, tobacco use, and diabetes we explored these relationships using our dataset and found the relative risk for each year of age was 1.07 (95% Confidence Interval 1.05-1.09; $p<0.001$), for each increase in BMI the odds ratio was 1.06 (95% Confidence Interval 1.02-1.09; $p<0.001$), for diabetes the odds ratio was 2.98 (95% Confidence Interval 1.79-4.98; $p<0.001$), and for tobacco use the odds ratio was 2.14 (95% Confidence Interval 1.21-3.79; $p<0.009$). When we adjusted for these risk factors there were no statistically significant differences in the Adjusted Odds Ratio for developing CHF for any of the developmental disabilities groups compared to those without disabilities.

One of the most important risk factors for the development of CHF is hypertension. The logistic regression derived odds ratio for CHF given hypertension was 7.15 (95% confidence interval 3.45-14.81, $p=0.001$). Thus we reran the adjusted odds ratio including hypertension and obtained the results shown in Table 3.

Table 1. Prevalence of having Congestive Heart Failure, among adults with no disability and those with developmental disability, by known risk factors

prevalence (ever)	without disability	All DD	Autism	Down syndrome	Cerebral Palsy	MR with Psychiatric Illness	MR
All	1809	694	54	58	163	152	267
	4.1	2.5	0.0	1.7	1.8	3.3	3.0
Gender							
Male	4.1	2.2	0.0	0.0	1.4	2.7	3.5
Female	4.1	2.8	0.0	4.1	2.3	3.9	2.5
Race							
White	3.2	2.7	0.0	2.3	1.9	4.0	3.3
African American	5.2	2.2	0.0	0.0	1.8	2.6	2.7
Other	0.0	0.0	0.0	0.0	0.0	0.0	0.0
Severity of Primary Disability							
Mild	n/a	n/a	0.0	0.0	4.0	4.4	5.1
Moderate	n/a	n/a	0.0	0.0	0.0	0.0	0.0
Severe	n/a	n/a	0.0	2.3	1.8	2.4	2.8
Residential Type							
Least Restrictive Environment	n/a	0.0	0.0	0.0	0.0	0.0	0.0
Most Restrictive Environment	n/a	1.9	0.0	6.3	3.5	0.0	1.3

Table 2. Adjusted* Odds Ratio for developing Congestive Heart Failure, by developmental disability group

Groups	n	Prevalence	Adjusted Odds Ratio	Lower Confidence Interval	Upper Confidence Interval	P-Value
Comparison	1809	4.1	1.00			
Autism	54	0.0				
Cerebral Palsy	163	1.7	1.90	0.54	6.71	0.321
Down syndrome	58	1.8	0.94	0.11	7.62	0.954
MR with Psychiatric Illness	152	3.3	1.38	0.52	3.65	0.520
MR Only	267	3.0	0.96	0.41	2.23	0.916

* adjusting for medical site, age, race, gender, BMI, tobacco use, and diabetes.

Table 3. Adjusted* Odds Ratio (with hypertension added) for developing Congestive Heart Failure, by developmental disability group

Groups	n	Prevalence	Adjusted Odds Ratio	Lower Confidence Interval	Upper Confidence Interval	P-Value
Comparison	1809	4.1	1.00			
Autism	54	0.0				
Cerebral Palsy	163	1.7	2.19	0.62	7.68	0.221
Down syndrome	58	1.8	1.43	0.17	11.77	0.741
MR with Psychiatric Illness	152	3.3	1.51	0.56	4.05	0.418
MR Only	267	3.0	1.12	0.48	2.62	0.787

*adjusting for medical site, age, race, gender, BMI, tobacco use, hypertension and diabetes.

Table 4. Adjusted* Odds Ratio for hypertension patients only for developing Congestive Heart Failure, by developmental disability group

Groups	n	Prevalence	Adjusted Odds Ratio	Lower Confidence Interval	Upper Confidence Interval	P-Value
Comparison	752	9.2	1.00			
Autism	8	0.0				
Cerebral Palsy	36	8.3	3.35	0.90	12.54	0.073
Down syndrome	10	0.0				
MR with Psychiatric Illness	55	7.3	1.42	0.47	4.31	0.540
MR Only	87	6.9	0.83	0.30	2.25	0.708

* adjusting for medical site, age, race, gender, BMI, tobacco use, and diabetes.

Again there was no group with statistically significant difference in prevalence of CHF compared to the comparison group, with hypertension included as a covariate. Finally, we stratified those with hypertension and looked at the odds of having CHF in Table 4.

In the model for hypertensive patients only the odds for having CHF for patients with cerebral palsy was marginally higher compared to the patients with hypertension but no disability.

We also explored the onset of CHF among those who entered the two practices without the condition, using Cox-proportional hazard modeling (survival analysis). In our dataset increases in starting BMI (Hazard Ratio 1.07; $p=0.001$) and development of diabetes (Hazard Ratio 1.98; $p=0.004$) were statistically significant associated with the onset of CHF. Then after controlling for these factors (BMI and diabetes) as well as age, race, BMI and tobacco use, there were no group differences in risk for onset of congestive heart failure. These results are shown in Table 5.

Table 5. Survival analysis, hazard ratio* of risk for Congestive Heart Failure, by risk group

Groups	N	Hazard Ratio	P-Value
Comparison	1803		
Autism	54		
Cerebral Palsy	163	1.05	0.930
Down syndrome	58	0.95	0.959
MR with Psychiatric Illness	152	0.97	0.947
MR Only	261	0.68	0.341

*controlling for medical site, race, gender, BMI, tobacco use and diabetes.

Implications from our study findings: It is important to acknowledge conditions with no significant difference between the sub-groups with developmental disabilities and the comparison group. Congestive heart failure falls into this category both in terms of disease prevalence and disease onset. In both cases the sub-groups with developmental disabilities were no different from the clinic patients without disability in terms of developing or living with CHF. However, we need to also recognize that both groups should be encouraged and assisted to reduce their risks for CHF though lifestyle change in diet and physical activity and control their co-morbid conditions.

Implications for Case Study: GM was a patient who was well liked by his peers, staff and physicians and his disturbing death left everyone feeling frustrated. He had early onset heart disease and a number of chronic health conditions. He took his medications and understood and tried to adhere to the lifestyle modifications suggested by his physician and staff. Nonetheless despite frequent physician visits the team was unsuccessful in reducing the trajectory of his decline and death. There is no real way to explain what went wrong and how his care could have been improved. There will always be a cause of death and until we can learn better ways to prevent and treat heart disease we can only say GM died of congestive heart failure.

References

Aronow WS. Heart Disease and Aging. *Med. Clin. North Am.,* 2006 90, 849-862.

Aronow WS, Ahn C, Kronzon I. Normal left ventricular ejection fraction in older persons with congestive heart failure. *Chest,* 1998 113, 867–869.

Aronow WS, Ahn C, Gutstein H. Prevalence and incidence of cardiovascular disease in 1160 older men and 2464 older women in a long-term health care facility. *J. Gerontol. A Biol. Sci. Med. Sci.,* 2002 57, 45–46.

Collins, RD. *Differential diagnosis in primary care.* 2003. Lippincott Williams and Wilkins.

Hayden MF. Mortality among people with mental retardation living in the United States: research review and policy application. *Mental. Retard.,* 1998 36, 345-359.

Kannel WB, Belanger AJ. Epidemiology of heart failure. *Am. Heart J.,* 1991 121, 951–957.

McDermott S, Moran R, Platt T, Wood H, Isaac T, Dasari S. Heart disease, schizophrenia and affective psychoses: epidemiology of risk in primary care. *Community Mental Health Journal,* 2005, 41, 747-55.

NHLBI. Congestive Heart Failure Data Fact Sheet, 1996. 2007 May 15. Available from: http://www.nhlbi_congestive_heart_failure_data_fact_sheet_nhlbi.htm.

NHLBI. Heart failure, 2007. 2007 June 8. Available from: http://www.nhlbi.nih.gov/health/dcl/Diseases/Hf/HF_Summary.html.

Patja K, Molsa P, Iivanainen M. Cause-specific mortality of people with intellectual disability in a population-based, 35-year follow-up study. *J. Intellect. Disabil. Res.,* 2001 45, 30-40.

van den Akker M, Maaskant MA, van der Meijden RJ. Cardiac diseases in people with intellectual disability. *J. Intellect. Disabil. Res.,* 2006 50, 515-522.

Chapter VII

Coronary Artery Disease

The Research Questions: What is the prevalence of coronary artery disease among adults with developmental disabilities and how does this compare to other adults, after controlling for known risk factors? For those adults who do not have coronary artery disease when they enter the family medicine practice sites under study, are there differences in the incidence of CAD for the impairment groups compared to those without a disability?

Definition of Coronary Artery Disease and Prevalence in the General Population: Coronary artery disease (CAD) occurs when the arteries that supply blood to the heart muscle (the coronary arteries) become hardened and narrowed due to buildup of plaque (atherosclerosis) on their inner walls. Eventually, blood flow to the heart muscle is reduced, and inadequate oxygen is supplied to the heart muscle resulting in:

- *Angina:* chest pain or discomfort that occurs when the heart doesn't get enough blood.
- *Heart attack (myocardial infarction):* when a blood clot develops at the site of plaque in a coronary artery and cuts off most or all blood supply to that part of the heart muscle causing permanent damage to the heart muscle.

Over time, CAD can weaken the heart muscle and contribute to:

- *Heart failure:* when the heart can't pump blood effectively to the rest of the body. *Arrhythmias:* changes in the normal beating rhythm of the heart.

CAD is the most common type of heart disease. It is the leading cause of death in the United States in both men and women (NHLBI et al, 2006).

Coronary artery disease (CAD) is one of the most common forms of heart disease. It is usually part of a systemic cardiovascular disease (CVD) – a narrowing of arteries in the heart and throughout the body over time due to atherosclerosis. This narrowing can significantly limit the amount of blood carried by the arteries and decrease the amount of oxygen supplied to the tissues. This can cause intermittent angina (chest pain) upon exercise. Unstable plaques are a major cause of heart attack (myocardial infarction) or other acute coronary syndrome. Dyspnea on exertion is a more common clinical manifestation of CAD in older men and women than is the typical chest pain of angina pectoris (Aronow et al, 2006).

Age is the highest risk factor for CAD and more than 83% of persons who die of CAD are aged 65 years or older (American Heart Association et al, 2007). The prevalence of CAD is similar in older women and men. Prospective epidemiologic studies have reported diabetes mellitus is an independent risk factor for the development of coronary artery disease and at coronary angiography or autopsy, diabetic patients have a higher incidence of double- and triple-vessel disease than do their non-diabetic counterparts (Grossman and Messerli et al, 1996; Orchard, Kretowski, Costacou, and Nesto et al, 2006). Diabetes mellitus and hypertension in the same patient have been shown to accelerate progression to more severe cardiomyopathy than would be expected with either condition alone (Grossmam and Messerli et al, 1996).

Literature Review of Coronary Artery Disease in Adults with Developmental Disability: Coronary Artery Disease and the risk factors associated with it have been studied in adults with developmental disabilities. Reports of decreased occurrence of CAD among individuals with Down syndrome contrasted with reports of increased occurrence among individuals with other genetic syndromes. In 1992 a study investigated the relationship of lipid and lipoprotein profiles in individuals with Down syndrome and the observed decreased occurrence of coronary artery disease. The results revealed triglyceride levels were significantly increased, and HDL cholesterol, apo AI and HDL cholesterol to total cholesterol ratio were significantly decreased in patients with Down syndrome when compared with the control group. No significant difference was observed between the study and control group with regard to total cholesterol, LDL cholesterol, apo B and the apo B to apo AI ratio. The observation of increased triglyceride levels and high HDL are usually associated with an increased risk for CAD, thus the decreased prevalence of coronary artery disease in the study individuals with Down syndrome could not be explained by the lipid and lipoprotein levels (Pueschel, Craig, and Haddow et al, 1992). More recently homocysteine metabolism has been studied in patients with Down syndrome because autosomal recessive inborn errors of metabolism, including cystathionine b-synthase (CBS) deficiency, is located on chromosome 21; homocysteine concentrations in Down syndrome are low because of the 3 copies of CBS (James, Pogribna, and Pogribny et al, 1999).

The prevalence of coronary artery disease among people with low prevalence genetic syndromes has also been studied. Premature arteriosclerosis has been reported in individuals with Prader-Willi, Turner's, Klinefelter, Cockayne, Werner syndromes and those with mitochondrial defects. Premature arteriosclerosis and elevated age-adjusted death rates were reported in adults with sex chromosome abnormalities such as Klinefelter and Turner's syndromes (Baker, Baba, and Boesel et al, 1981). Many of these syndromes have been reported as having higher risk for diabetes, hyperlipidemia, hypertension, and obesity and all of these factors are associated with increased risk for coronary artery disease (Wallace et al, 2004).

What is the Conceptual Framework for this question?: The notion of normalcy in the community integration of people with developmental disabilities leads us to question whether people with DD have a different risk for onset of coronary artery disease compared to their peers without disability. If in fact people with DD have similar lifestyles and risk factors as the general population then we would expect difference in their profile for CAD to be explained by factors related to their disability status. However, it is thought that people with DD have lower rates of smoking, even if their diet and physical activity are not entirely different from the general population, and this might lower their risk. Our study allows us to explore likenesses and differences between the groups so we can begin to understand some of these issues.

Case Study: CS is a 54 year old white male with moderate mental retardation (ICD9 318.0) who has had a long history of hypertension (ICD9 401.9) treated by Dr. E. with lisinopril (Prinivil) and hydrochlorothiazide (Microzide). Dr. E. first saw CS in his family medicine practice 15 years ago when at the age of 39 he had already established hypertension and hyperlipidemia (ICD9 272.0). The hyperlipidemia is presently being treated with atorvastatin calcium (Lipitor).

Six years ago CS developed diabetes mellitus (ICD9 250.00) and is presently on metformin (Glucophage) and glipizide (Glucotrol). His other medical conditions include GERD (ICD9 350.81) being treated with esomeprazole sodium (Nexium) 40 mg per day and hypothyroidism (ICD9 244.9) being treated with replacement therapy. CS lives in a community training home (CTH) II.

Over the last four years Dr. E. noted CS's weight has fluctuated between 192 and 215 which for his height of 5'7" results in BMI's between 30 and 34. And despite efforts at instruction by Dr. E and his nursing staff related to establishing a habit for taking his medication, referral to weight management programs, encouraging and actually prescribing physical activity goals CS's blood pressure and glucose have been poorly controlled at times. This has resulted in part from CS's failure to regularly take his medications as prescribed and his binge eating habits.

One year ago CS had an episode of chest pains while walking from the bus into the workshop which is part of his daily activity. He was taken to the local hospital where he was found to have acute changes on his EKG and he was then taken to the Cardiac catherization laboratory were he had two stints placed in his right coronary artery and his circumflex artery. He has subsequently done well except for an occasional episode of chest pain. CS has returned to his previous level of activity; however his diabetes, hypertension, and weight have proven difficult to control.

Our Research Findings: We identified a 7 percent prevalence of coronary artery disease among the patients without disability in our two practices. All the groups with developmental disabilities had substantially lower rates, ranging from no cases of CAD among patients with autism and Down syndrome to a prevalence rate of 3.8 percent for patients with mental retardation (Table 1).

Table 1. Prevalence of Coronary Artery Disease by disability status, and risk factors

prevalence (ever)	without disability	All DD	Autism	Down Syndrome	Cerebral Palsy	MR with Psychiatric Illness	MR
All	1809	694	54	58	163	152	267
	6.9	2.0	No cases	No cases	1.2	1.3	3.8
Gender							
Male	8.1	2.2	0.0	0.0	2.7	0.0	4.1
Female	6.0	1.9	0.0	0.0	0.0	2.6	3.3
Race							
White	9.0	2.2	0.0	0.0	1.9	1.3	3.9
African American	5.4	1.8	0.0	0.0	0.0	1.3	3.6
Other	0.0	0.0	0.0	0.0	0.0	0.0	0.0
Severity of Primary Disability							
Mild	n/a	n/a	0.0	0.0	2.0	2.2	4.1
Moderate	n/a	n/a	0.0	0.0	1.8	0.0	3.3
Severe	n/a	n/a	0.0	0.0	0.0	0.0	3.7
Residential Type							
Least Restrictive Environment	n/a	0.0	0.0	0.0	0.0	0.0	0.0
Most Restrictive Environment	n/a	1.5	0.0	0.0	1.7	0.0	66.7

Table 2. Logistic Regression* Odds Ratios for Risk of Coronary Artery Disease, by developmental disability group

Groups	n	Prev.	Adjusted* Odds Ratio	Lower Confidence Interval	Upper Confidence Interval	P-Value
Comparison	1809	6.9	1.00			
Autism	54	0.0	No cases			
Cerebral Palsy	163	0.0	0.47	0.10	2.14	0.328
Down syndrome	58	1.2	No cases			
MR with Psychiatric Illness	152	1.3	0.25	0.06	1.06	0.060
MR Only	267	3.8	0.73	0.35	1.55	0.417

*controlling for medical site, age, race, gender, BMI, diabetes, and tobacco use.

Since some risk factors are well established in their association with CAD we explore the risk factors of age, race, gender, diabetes and tobacco use in our study population. Each year of age was associated with an 8 percent increase in risk: Odds Ratio 1.08; 95% Confidence Interval 1.06-1.11, p=0.001. Both diabetes and tobacco use were associated with a three fold increase in risk for coronary artery disease: OR 3.64; (2.30-5.76), p=0.001 and OR 3.20; (1.96-5.22), p=0.001, respectively. When we performed logistic regression adjusting for these risk factors there was no statistically significant difference in the risk for CAD in any of the developmental disabilities groups compared to the comparison patients (Table 2). Patients with mental retardation and psychiatric illness have a marginally significant lower risk for CAD compared to those without disabilities (Adjusted Odds Ratio 0.25, p=0.06).

Finally, we looked at the onset of CAD among the individuals in the groups who did not have CAD when they entered the practices for care. Again, we explored the known risk factors and found a statistically significant risk associated with being male (Hazard Rate 1.72; p=0.004), white (Hazard Rate 1.61; p=0.019), having a higher starting BMI (Hazard Rate 1.03; p=0.029), having diabetes (Hazard Rate 2.24; p=0.001), and being a smoker (Hazard Rate 2.05; p=0.001). When we controlled for all of these confounders the risk of onset of CAD was statistically significantly lower for the MR group (Hazard Ratio 0.50, p=0.05) and for the group with MR and psychiatric illness (Hazard Ratio 0.20, p=0.03), compared to those with no disability. For patients with cerebral palsy there was no difference in the onset rate compared to those without disabilities. These results are shown in Table 3.

Table 3. Survival analysis, Hazard Ratio for onset of coronary artery disease, by group

Groups	n	Hazard Ratio	P-Value
Comparison	1799		
Autism	54	No cases	
Cerebral Palsy	163	0.37	0.165
Down syndrome	58	No cases	
MR with Psychiatric Illness	152	**0.22**	**0.034**
MR Only	261	**0.50**	**0.049**

* controlling for medical site, age, race, gender, BMI, diabetes, and tobacco use.
Bold indicates statistically significant.

Implications from our study findings: First of all we cannot say anything about the risk for coronary artery disease for adults with autism or Down syndrome since we had a small number of individuals in these groups (approximately 55 per group) and there were no cases of CAD. The survival analysis results in Table 3 suggest that people with mental retardation with or without psychiatric disease were statistically significantly less likely to develop CAD it they came to the practice without established CAD. When we include those with established CAD when they entered the study sites the Odds Ratio for people with MR was not statistically significantly different from the comparison group (Table 2). Thus overall there was no difference in the prevalence of CAD but in our practices adults with MR, with and without psychiatric illness, who entered care without CAD were statistically significantly less likely to develop CAD than their counterparts without disabilities during the years of follow-up at these family medicine sites.

Implications for Case Study: CS is not an unusual patient in the primary care practice in his uneven adjustment to his chronic conditions and his compulsion to overeat. Maintaining a consistent relationship with his health care providers has allowed for continuity in one arena of his life where many factors have been changing. Residential staff in group setting for adults with developmental disability, do not have a history of longevity in their employment and the staff at the workshop where CS spends his weekdays has also fluctuated. It is not unexpected that hypertension and diabetes are difficult to control and require regular monitoring. The additional challenge of monitoring the individual with coronary artery disease include concerns about poly-pharmacy, regular attention to promotion of health through education about choices, and providing encouragement to be physically active and eat healthy foods.

References

Aronow WS. Heart disease and aging. *Med. Clin. North Am.*, 2006 90, 849-62.

Baker PB, Baba N, Boesel CP. Cardiovascular abnormalities in progeria. Case report and review of the literature. *Arch. Pathol. Lab. Med.*, 1981 105, 384-6.

Grossman E, Messerli FH. Diabetic and Hypertensive Heart Disease. *Ann. Intern. Med*, 1996 125, 304-10.

James JS, Pogribna M, Pogribny IP, et al. Abnormal folate metabolism and mutation in the methylenetetrahydrofolate reductase gene may be maternal risk factors for Down syndrome. *Am. J. Clin. Nutr.*, 1999 70, 495-501.

Orchard TJ, Kretowski A, Costacou T, Nesto RW. Type 1 Diabetes and Coronary Artery Disease. *Diabetes care*, 2006 29, 2528-38.

Pueschel SM, Craig WY, Haddow JE. Lipids and lipoproteins in persons with Down's syndrome. *J. Intellect Disabil. Res*, 1992 35, 365-9.

Wallace RA. Risk factors for Coronary Artery Disease among Individuals with Rare Syndrome Intellectual Disabilities. *Journal of Policy and Practice in Intellectual Disabilities*, 2004 1, 42-51.

Chapter VIII

Depression

The Research Questions: What is the prevalence of depression among adults with developmental disabilities and how does this compare to other adults without disabilities, after controlling for established risk characteristics? For those adults who do not have depression when they enter the family medicine practice sites under study, are there differences in the incidence of depression among the impairment groups compared to those without a disability?

Definition of Depression and Prevalence in the General Population: The Diagnostic and Statistical Manual of Mental Disorders (DSM-IV) lists depressive disorders under Mood Disorders. Included in this category are major depressive disorder, dysthymic disorder, bipolar disorder, cyclothymic disorder, mood disorder due to a general medical condition, and substance-induced mood disorder. For each of these mood disorders there are specific criteria about symptoms that must be met to receive the diagnosis. Specifiers associated with the mood disorders are level of the condition (mild, moderate, severe), presence of psychotic features, recurrence and remission, chronicity, and presence of features (catatonic, melancholic, atypical, with full inter-episode recovery, seasonal pattern, rapid-cycling) (American Psychiatric Association et al, 1994).

Lifetime prevalence rates for depression in community-based surveys range from 5 to 15%. (Kessler, McGonagle, and Zhoa, et al, 1994; Chen, Eaton, Gallo, Nestadt and Crum et al, 2000; Kessler, Berglund, Demler, and Jin et al, 2003; Riolo, Nguyen, Greden, and King et al, 2005) The wide range in the prevalence estimates is related to the use of different ascertainment methods, ranging from use of screening questionnaires to determining if people have received a diagnosis based on review of medical records. We would expect screening questionnaires to pick up more people with depression compared findings from a review of medical records in primary care sites. In addition, even when a screening instrument is used the site of screening (medical versus community) would contribute to the prevalence estimates. Finally the choice of a screening instrument will impact prevalence estimates since the instruments have different sensitivity and specificity.

Risk factors for depression include gender (two to three fold increased risk for women), age (decade of life and cohort effects), urban-rural residence (higher in urban areas), marital status (married and never-divorced had the lowest rates), family history (two to three fold increased risk among first-degree relatives), and socioeconomic status (unemployment and poverty are associated with higher risk) (Horwarth and Weissman et al, 1995; Everson, Maty, Lynch, and Kaplan et al, 2002). Thus, depending on where a study is carried out and the methods used for ascertainment, the reported rates among groups have varied.

Literature Review of Depression in Adults with Developmental Disability: Mental health problems in adults with developmental disabilities have been studied since the 1980s (Sturmey and Sevin et al, 1993). The majority of research has concentrated on describing the clinical manifestation of depression in this group (Charlot, Doucette, and Mezzacappa et al, 1993; Meins et al, 1995; Davis, Judd, and Herman et al, 1997; Marston, Perry, and Roy et al, 1997). A 2003 review of assessment and diagnosis methods for people with developmental disability reports "for those with mild to moderate intellectual disability, a consensus is emerging that standard diagnostic criteria are appropriate" but for people with severe and profound intellectual disability there is debate about diagnostic criteria (McBrien et al, 2003). Although there is variability in prevalence rates of depression, depending on the methodology, depression was identified or diagnosed in 25-44% of individuals with developmental disability, in most studies. (Marston, Perry, and Roy et al, 1997; McBrien et al, 2003) As described for the general population this range in prevalence rates is in part based on the ascertainment method, the setting for the case finding, and variability in other methods used in the studies.

It has been reported that mental illness occurs in about 30 percent of persons with Down syndrome. Using Diagnostic Research Criteria (DCR-10) depression, obsessive-compulsive disorder, and conduct disorder are the most common diagnoses for this group (Prasher et al, 1995). It has been suggested that depression is three times more common in people with Down syndrome than in people with other types of mental retardation (Chicoine, McGuire, and Rubin et al, 1999; Cooper and Collacott al, 1994). In the largest study of community dwelling adults with Down syndrome in the United Kingdom 11.1% had experienced at last one depressive episode when the DSM-III-R criteria were used. The average age of onset of depression was 29 years and women were more likely than men to experience an episode. (Cooper and Collacott et al, 1994).

Individuals with autism also have been reported to demonstrate symptoms of a number of co-morbid mental illness conditions including affective disorders. The most frequent co-morbid diagnoses for adults with autism are mood and anxiety disorders and there are research reports that there is a higher rate of depression in individuals with autism. Because many individuals with autism do not have the verbal skills to describe their symptoms, clinicians must be sensitive to nonverbal signs of depression (Ghaziuddin, Ghaziuddin, and Greden et al, 2002).

What is the Conceptual Framework for this question?: The epidemiology of mental illness among people with developmental disabilities has been studied for decades. The overall prevalence of mental illness among this subpopulation is thought to be substantially higher than expected for the general population, however, the contribution of genetic predisposition and the impact of risk factors related to lifestyle challenges is not well established.

For the most part people with developmental disabilities live in the community and have both opportunities and challenges to participation in many aspects of adult life. Adults with developmental disabilities have regular exposure to people without disabilities who are not in a caregiver role and there are venues for socialization in both integrated and segregated settings. However, most adults with cognitive disabilities have restricted social networks and they also often fall into a high risk group for depression based on unemployment and poverty. The impact of these social and environmental risks combined with biologic (genetic and acquired) factors could contribute to high rates of depression in adults with developmental disabilities.

Case Study: CC is a 53 year old Caucasian male with moderate mental retardation (ICD9 318), cerebral palsy with spastic quadriplegia (ICD9 343.2) and seizure disorder (ICD9 780.39). He has a limited vocabulary and is difficult to understand. In addition, he uses a wheelchair for mobility. Two years ago he was required to move away from his family home and community due to his mother's failing health and subsequent death. CC was moved to a community where his lone surviving sibling, a sister lived and he was placed in an ICF MR Community residence. At this time CC joined the practice of Dr. P. who provided care to the residents of the ICF through a contract with the local disability agency.

Soon after arrival at his residence the staff told Dr. P. that CC's behavior was disruptive if he did not get something that he wanted. He would scream, thrash in his wheelchair or bed, and he had great difficulty getting calm again. Approximately six months after he moved in the residence CC had lost 15 pounds and his BMI was 20. In addition, CC wanted more time alone in his room and the staff began reporting episodes of head banging and compulsive scratching on his leg. Dr. P; referred CC's to a psychiatrist who had substantial experience working with adults with mental retardation. He received a diagnosis of depression (ICD9 311) and was placed on a selective serotonin reuptake inhibitor (SSRI) anti-depressant. Staff and family were informed of his depressive diagnosis and he started seeing a psychiatrist on a regular basis for medication adjustments and monitoring of his condition. After his depression diagnosis staff and family tried to be more attentive and understanding to CC's emotional situation. After several months on his SSRI it was noted that he seemed to have fewer episodes of self abuse or disruptive behavior and CC was participating in more activities with his housemates. Dr. P. agreed to assume responsibility for follow-up and medication adjustment, with annual visits to the psychiatrist.

Our Research Findings: We used medical records to identify diagnosed cases of depression. The listing of any of the following ICD-9 codes: 300.4, 311, 296.2, 296.3 or 309.1 were used to identify potential cases of depression from the medical record. There was substantial variation in the use of codes by the numerous providers in the two practices, over the average of ten years of care for most of the patients, thus the case definition of depression could only be met if in addition to identifying an ICD9 code in the medical record, a diagnosis of depression was verified in the progress notes, problem lists, or consultation note from a psychiatrist or psychologist (McDermott, Moran, Platt, Issac, Wood, and Dasari et al, 2005).

The overall prevalence of depression in the comparison patients (24%) was significantly different from the prevalence in the patients with developmental disability (17%; p=0.0184). Among the people with developmental disabilities, the prevalence of depression was lowest in the group with autism (4%) and highest among those with MR and psychiatric illness (26%). The later category, MR with psychiatric illness, includes those with major depression so we would expect this group to have the highest prevalence rate.

In order to do multiple variable modeling we explored the prevalence of depression by risk factors for each of the groups. As expected women were more likely than men to be diagnosed with depression, whites were more likely than African-Americans to have the diagnosis, and milder forms of developmental disability and less restrictive community home living were associated with higher rates. Each of these risk factors was statistically significantly associated with depression. In fact being female was associated with an adjusted Odds Ratio of 2.7 (95% Confidence Interval 2.2-3.4, p=0.001) and being African-American had a protective effect with only half the risk for depression compared to whites (Adjusted Odds Ratio 0.5: 95% Confidence Interval 0.4-0.6, p=0.001). We also looked at smoking status and found that smokers had elevated odds for depression (Adjusted Odds Ratio 1.7: 95% Confidence Interval 1.3-2.1, p=0.001).

After controlling for the known risk factors, three groups, those with autism (Adjusted Odds Ratio 0.18: 95% Confidence Interval 0.04- 0.74, p=0.02), cerebral palsy (Adjusted Odds Ratio 0.6: 95% Confidence Interval 0.38- 0.96, p=0.03), and those with MR (Adjusted Odds Ratio 0.68: 95% Confidence Interval 0.48- 0.97, p=0.03) had a statistically significant lower risk for depression compared to patients without disability. This is shown in Table 2.

We also explored the relationship between severity of the primary disabling condition and depression to determine if the groups with mild, moderate and severe primary disabilities had different rates and odds for depression. The unadjusted percent of people in the study groups with depression, by the severity of their developmental disability, is shown in Table 3. We then did logistic regression, shown in Table 4, and it demonstrates individuals with mild developmental disabilities did not differ from the comparison group in their odds ratio for depression. However, the adults with a moderate level of autism, both moderate and severe cerebral palsy, and severe level of MR had odds ratios that were protective for depression.

We used survival analysis to show the onset of depression for patients who were free of depression when they entered the study sites for care. Again, we assessed the risk for depression for each of the risk factors and found statistically significant risk groups. The hazard ratio for women compared to men was 2.0 (p=0.001), for African-American compared to whites it was 0.69 (p=0.001), and for smokers it was 1.36 (p=0.002). Table 5 shows there were no statistically significant differences in the incidence of depression in the patients with developmental disabilities compared to patients without disabilities.

Table 1. Unadjusted Prevalence of depression by disability status for risk groups

prevalence (ever)	Without disability	All DD	Autism	Down syndrome	Cerebral Palsy	MR with Psychiatric Illness	MR
All	1809	694	54	58	163	152	267
	23.7	16.7	3.7	12.1	14.7	26.3	16.1
Gender							
Male	14.5	13.0	4.8	8.8	12.2	17.6	14.5
Female	30.9	20.9	0.0	16.7	16.9	34.6	18.0
Race							
White	29.1	19.5	5.3	14.0	17.9	33.3	19.0
African American	19.2	12.5	0.0	7.1	8.9	19.5	11.8
Other	14.6	0.0	0.0	0.0	0.0	0.0	0.0
Severity of Primary Disability							
Mild	n/a	n/a	0.0	33.3	26.0	27.8	24.5
Moderate	n/a	n/a	5.1	12.5	8.9	28.6	23.3
Severe	n/a	n/a	0.0	9.1	10.5	22.0	4.6
Residential Type							
Least Restrictive Environment	n/a	25.0	33.3	25.0	10.0	47.8	20.4
Most Restrictive Environment	n/a	14.6	6.3	12.5	8.6	25.0	16.3

Table 2. Logistic Regression Adjusted* Odds Ratio for depression by disability group

Groups	n	Prev.	Adjusted Odds Ratio	Lower Confidence Interval	Upper Confidence Interval	P-Value
Comparison	1809	23.7	1.00			
Autism	54	3.7	**0.18**	**0.04**	**0.74**	**0.018**
Cerebral Palsy	163	12.1	**0.60**	**0.38**	**0.96**	**0.032**
Down syndrome	58	14.7	0.50	0.22	1.14	0.100
MR with Psychiatric Illness	152	26.3	1.21	0.82	1.80	0.332
MR Only	267	16.1	**0.68**	**0.48**	**0.97**	**0.034**

*adjusting for medical site, age, gender, race, and smoking status.
Bold indicates statistically significantly different from comparison patients.

Table 3. Comparison of percent with depression, by severity of developmental disability

Severity of condition	Mild	Moderate	Severe
Autism	-	5.1	-
Down syndrome	33.3	12.5	9.1
Cerebral Palsy	26.0	8.9	10.5
MR with psychiatric Illness	27.8	28.6	22.0
MR Only	24.5	23.3	4.6

Table 4. Adjusted* Odds Ratio for depression by severity of developmental disability

Groups	Adjusted Odds Ratio	Lower Confidence Interval	Upper Confidence Interval	P-Value
Mild developmental disability versus comparison group				
Comparison	1.00			
Autism				0.957
Cerebral Palsy	1.24	0.64	2.41	0.525
Down syndrome	1.36	0.24	7.69	0.731
MR with Psychiatric Illness	1.29	0.78	2.11	0.319
MR Only	1.01	0.62	1.65	0.959
Moderate developmental disability versus comparison group				
Comparison	1.00			
Autism	**0.24**	**0.06**	**1.02**	**0.054**
Cerebral Palsy	**0.36**	**0.14**	**0.93**	**0.035**
Down syndrome	0.64	0.07	5.50	0.681
MR with Psychiatric Illness	1.47	0.54	3.98	0.452
MR Only	1.13	0.60	2.13	0.705
Severe developmental disability versus comparison group				
Comparison	1.00			
Autism				0.977
Cerebral Palsy	**0.35**	**0.15**	**0.84**	**0.019**
Down syndrome	0.37	0.13	1.04	0.060
MR with Psychiatric Illness	0.95	0.44	2.06	0.887
MR Only	**0.18**	**0.07**	**0.46**	**0.000**

*controlling for medical site, age, gender, race, and smoking status.
Bold indicates statistically significantly different from comparison patients.

Table 5. Survival Analysis* Hazard Rates for developing depression, by subgroup

Groups	n	Hazard Ratio	P-Value
Comparison	1748		
Autism	54	0.40	0.192
Cerebral Palsy	159	0.82	0.383
Down syndrome	58	0.64	0.278
MR with Psychiatric Illness	140	0.99	0.944
MR Only	252	0.78	0.138

*controlling for medical site, age, gender, race, and smoking status.

Implications from Our Study Findings: The limitations of our study include reliance on physician diagnosis of depression without the use of standardized assessment instruments, the small sample size for some of the case groups, and the retrospective identification of the case and comparison groups. However, the use of a retrospective cohort allowed more complete ascertainment of depression because of repeated contacts with the primary care physician. This is important because our study group came from a community population, not from specialty clinics, disability service providers, or persons living in institutions, often used in epidemiology studies. Other studies rely on a cross-sectional sample where there is potential to include patients with a history of circumstantial depression who are maintained on medications for many years, resulting in over-identification of depression (McDermott, Moran, Platt, Issac, Wood and Dasari et al, 2005).

Primary care providers are often criticized for under-diagnosing depression. In a study of over 1800 primary care adult patients 30% had high levels of depression symptoms when the Duke Health Profile was administered, however only 5% had the diagnosis listed in their medical record. In our study we relied on the diagnosis of depression in the medical record and thus, we probably underestimated the problem in both the case and the comparison groups. The discrepancy between screened rates and diagnosed rates in primary care settings results from a variety of issues including diagnostic overshadowing of psychiatric and medical symptoms and the short encounter time for most ambulatory care encounters (Wu, Parkerson, and Doraiswamy et al, 2002). The limitation of using the medical diagnoses of depression rather than screening with standardized instruments is there could be under identification of depression in patients with severe disabilities, since it is difficult to recognize signs of depression in these individuals. However, disability researchers have faulted studies that rely on standardized assessment instruments which might not be understood by individuals with cognitive disabilities. In the field of disability research, there is also concern that case ascertainment methods in community based studies are biased against individuals with disabilities because recruitment of these adults is not a priority. Disability researchers have used self report, interviews and medical records to report depression prevalence (McDermott, Moran, Platt, Issac, Wood, and Dasari et al, 2005).

Additional research is needed to determine whether these results generalize to other settings. In this study there was no difference in the prevalence of depression among the patients with and without developmental disabilities and there was lower incidence for those who were depression free when they enrolled in the practices (McDermott, Moran, Platt, Issac, Wood, and Dasari et al, 2005).

Implications for Case Study: The field of duel diagnosis, mental retardation and mental illness, has emerged as a specialty in psychiatry and most state programs serving individuals with developmental disabilities employ a psychiatrist. Clearly the needs of people with developmental disabilities are somewhat different from the psychiatric needs of those without a disability so special training is usually needed to provide comprehensive psychiatric services. In the case of CC the family medicine physician has established a close working relationship with a psychiatrist who specialized in adults with DD. Together they are able to prevent poly-pharmacy and they communicate about concerns and issues as they arise.

References

Charlot L, Doucette A, Mezzacappa E. Affective symptoms of institutionalized adults with mental retardation. *Am. J. Ment. Retar.,* 1993 98, 408-416.

Chen LS, Eaton WW, Gallo JJ, Nestadt G, Crum RM. Empirical examination of current depression categories in a population-based study: symptoms, course, and risk factors. *Am. J. Psychiarty,* 2000 157, 573-580.

Chicoine, B; McGuire, D; Rubin, SS. Specialty clinic perspectives. In: Janicki MP, Dalton AJ, eds. *Dementia, aging, and intellectual disabilities: a handbook.* Philadelphia: Brunner/Mazel; 1999; 278-93.

Cooper SA, Collacott RA. Clinical features and diagnostic criteria of depression in Down's syndrome. *Br. J. Psychiatry,* 1994 165, 399–403.

Davis J, Judd F, Herman H. Depression in adults with intellectual disability. Part 1: A review. Australian and New Zealand *Journal of Psychiatry,* 1997 31, 232-242.

Everson SA, Maty SC, Lynch JW, Kaplan GA. Epidemiologic evidence for the relation between socioeconomic status and depression, obesity, and diabetes. *Journal of Psychosomatic Research,* 2002 53, 891-895.

Ghaziuddin M, Ghaziuddin N, Greden J. Depression in persons with autism: implications for research and clinical care. *J. of Autism and Developmental Disorders,* 2002, 32, 4, 299-306.

Horwath E, Weissman M. Epidemiology of depression and anxiety disorders. In: Tsuang M, Tohen M, Zahner G. *Textbook in psychiatric epidemiology.* New York: Wiley and Sons, Inc.; 1995; 317-344.

Kessler RC, Berglund P, Demler O, Jin R, Koretz D, Merikangas KR, Rush AJ, Walters EE, Wang PS, National Comorbidity Survey Replication. The epidemiology of major depressive disorder: results for the National Comorbidity Survey Replication (NCS-R). *JAMA,* 2003 289, 3095-3105.

Kessler, RC; McGonagle, KA; Zhoa S. Lifetime and 12-month prevalence of DSM-III-R psychiatric disorders in the United States. Results from the National Comorbidity Survey. *Arch. Gen. Psychiarty.*1994 51, 8-19.

Marston G, Perry D, Roy A. Manifestations of depression in people with intellectual disability. *J. Intellect. Disabil. Res.,* 1997 41, 476-480.

McBrien, JA. Assessment and diagnosis of depression in people with intellectual disability. *J. Intellect. Disabil. Res.,* 2003 47, 1-13.

McDermott, S; Moran, R; Platt, T; Issac, T; Wood, H; Dasari S. Depression in adults with disabilities, in primary care. *Disabilities and Rehabilitation,* 2005 7, 117-123.

Meins W. Symptoms of major depression in mentally retarded adults. *J. Intellect. Disabil. Res.,* 1995 39, 41-45.

Prasher, VP. Prevalence of psychiatric disorders in adults with Down syndrome. *Eur. J. Psyc.,* 1995 9, 77-82.

Pignone, MP; Gaynes, BN; Rushton, JL. Screening for Depression in Adults: A Summary of the Evidence. *Ann. Intern. Me,* 2002 136, 765-776.

Riolo, SA, Nguyen TA, Greden JF, King CA. Prevalence of depression by race/ethnicity: findings from the National Health and Nutrition Examination Survey III. *Am. J. of Public Health,* 2005.

Sturmey P, Sevin J. Dual diagnosis: an annotated bibliography of resent research. *J. Intellect. Disabil. Res.,* 1993 3,408-416. , 95, 6, 998-1000.

Wu L, Parkerson G, Doraiswamy P. Health perception, pain, and disability as correlates of anxiety and depression symptoms in primary care patients. *J. Am. Board Fam. Pract.,* 2002 15, 183-190.

Chapter IX

Dementia

The Research Questions: What is the prevalence of dementia among adults with developmental disabilities and how does this compare to other adults, after controlling for known risk factors? For those adults who do not have dementia when they enter the family medicine practice sites under study, are there differences in the incidence of dementia among the impairment groups compared to those without a disability?

Definition of Dementia and Prevalence in the General Population: Dementia is a neurodegenerative disease with progressive decline in cognitive function due to damage or disease in the brain beyond what might be expected from normal aging. The most common form of dementia is Alzheimer's disease (AD) however the only definite way to diagnose AD is to find out whether there are plaques and tangles in brain tissue at autopsy. Therefore a diagnosis of possible or probable AD can only be made while the person is alive so dementia is often used to cover both dementia and AD.

The brain functions that are substantially impacted by dementia are memory, attention, language, and problem solving. Especially in the later stages of the condition, affected persons may be disoriented in time, in place, and in person (Bird and Miller et al, 2007). Dementia it is characterized by progressive cognitive deterioration resulting in increasing dependence on others for activities of daily living and behavior changes. The most striking early symptom is amnesia, manifested as forgetfulness that becomes steadily more pronounced, with relative preservation of older memories. As the disorder progresses, cognitive impairment extends to the domains of language (aphasia), skilled movements (apraxia), recognition (agnosia), and functions closely related to the frontal and temporal lobes of the brain as they become disconnected from the limbic system. The pathologic process consists of neuronal loss or atrophy in the temporoparietal cortex and the frontal cortex, together with an inflammatory response to the deposition of amyloid plaques and neurofibrillary tangles (Med Track Alert et al, 2007).

Three to 11 percent of persons over 65 years of age, and 25% to 47% of those older than 85 years of age have been reported to have dementia (U.S. Office of Technology Assessment et al, 1987; Evans and Funkenstein, et al, 1989; Evans, Smith, Scherr, Albert, Funkenstein and Hebert et al, 1991; U.S. General Accounting Office et al, 1998; Patterson, Gauthier,

Bergman, Cohen, Feightner, and Feldman et al, 1999; McDowell, Hill, Lindsay, and Helliwell et al, 1994). It is apparent that the incidence of dementia is highest in the seventh and eighth decades of life resulting in high prevalence rates among people who survivor to this age.

Research in primary care settings among patients older than 65 years of age indicates approximately six percent have dementia, but approximately 50% have not received a diagnosis (O'Connor, Pollitt, Hyde, Brook, Reiss, and Roth et al, 1988; Lagaay, van der Meij, and Hijmans et al, 1992; Cooper, Bickel, and Schaufele et al, 1996; Olafsdottir, Skoog, and Marcusson et al, 2000; Valcour, Masaki, Curb, and Blanchette et al, 2000). According to the US Preventive Services Task Force clinicians who rely on routine history taking and physical examination often miss the opportunity to diagnose dementia during clinic visits (Boustani, Peterson, Hanson, Harris, and Lohr et al, 2003).

Literature Review of Dementia in Adults with Developmental Disability: Large population studies show that the rate of occurrence of dementia among persons with mental retardation and related developmental disabilities does not substantially differ from the general population incidence rate (Janicki and Dalton et al, 2000). However there is substantial evidence that people with Down syndrome have extremely high rates of Alzheimer's disease and a growing body of research suggests that almost all persons with Down syndrome over age 35-40 show the signs of Alzheimer's disease. When autopsy is conducted nearly all older adults with Down syndrome show the brain changes associated with Alzheimer's disease (Zigman, Schupf, Zigman, Silverman et al, 1993; Wherret et al, 1999). Down syndrome accounts for approximately 8-10% of people with mental retardation and the rate of dementia among adults with Down syndrome are as high as 55% in persons aged 40-50 years, and 75% in persons aged 60 years and older (Lai and Williams et al, 1989).

The onset and course of the disease in this group are atypical and may be more problematic because adults with Down syndrome are younger when affected (Visser, Aldenkamp, van Huffelen, Kuilman, Overweg, and van Wijk et al, 1997) and, in some instances, experience a more rapid disease-related decline in function (Janicki and Dalton et al, 1999). The disease course generally mirrors that of other people, although individuals with Down syndrome experience earlier appearances of personality changes, losses in mental abilities, losses in memory, and seizures; about 19% of adults with Down syndrome were reported to have late onset seizures (Janicki and Dalton et al, 2000). There are specific guidelines in place for the identification and care of people with intellectual disability and Alzheimer's disease (Janicki, Heller, Seltzer, and Hogg et al, 1996). These guidelines were developed to encourage guidance for management and for training and education of caregivers. In adults with Down syndrome the average age of onset is in the 50's, with death likely to occur between 2 to 7 years after onset (Janicki and Dalton et al, 2000). There is no other known subset of people with developmental disabilities with elevated risk for dementia.

What is the Conceptual Framework for this question?: The double blow to reduced cognitive function associated with dementia developing among adults with Down syndrome brings the affected group to a markedly compromised functional status. In addition, although the other developmental disability groups might not have statistically significantly different prevalence of dementia compared to the general population it is important to assess the magnitude of the problem for these groups, as well.

The need for additional supports and the implications for caregivers are important issues, as the life span increases and the added disability associated with dementia is manifest. Our study of both prevalence and incidence is important since it has implications for program and policy development in the field of disability services. We need information about the magnitude of challenges associated with dementia for adults with DD.

Case Study: HG was a 51 year old female with Down syndrome (ICD9 758.00) and hyperthyroidism (ICD9 244.9) who was high functioning despite a diagnostic level of moderate mental retardation (ICD9 318.0). She lived for approximately 10 years in a CTH in the community, with frequent returns to her family home where her parents and younger sister lived. During this period HG began what became a long term relationship with her family physician Dr. P.

At age 53 Dr. P. noted substantial changes in her mental status resulting in diminished awareness of her surroundings and greater reliance on support staff. Dr. P. administered a mental status examination and concluded HG was starting to develop the symptoms of Alzheimer's disease. Dr. P. talked with HG's family and direct support staff about the increased concerns for her safety and the need to provide close supervision during outings. He also counseled the family and staff to be alert to mood changes and to keep notes on behaviors and issues that concerned them. Over the next two to three years HGs dementia progressed quite rapidly despite many added supports and the use of both donepezil hydrochloride (Aricept) and memantine hydrochloride (Namenda) prescribed by Dr. P. The notes and verbal reports to Dr. P. indicated her family and staff saw no clinical response to these medications, and the progression of the Alzheimers continued at a rapid pace.

By age 55 years HG used a wheelchair for mobility and spent protracted periods in bed and in the house. Staff reported she now required essentially total care and within a year HG moved back to an ICF MR level of care. HG's elderly parents and younger sister asked for a consultation with Dr. P. during this period of rapid functional decline and they opted to have a PEG placed after long discussions with her personal care staff, as well as Dr. P.. Over the next 3 years HG become progressively more disabled and had very limited ability to interact with her environment. She developed small, frequent seizures (ICD9 780.39) episodes which were treated with carbamazepine (Tegretol) and valporic acid (Depakene). In addition, she had at least one hospitalization for aspiration related to pneumonia (ICD9 507.8). Her mental functioning continued to deteriorate to the point that she was barely able to be aroused and she remained in this state for over 6 months.

Again Dr. P. had multiple conversations with her family and support staff, and then arranged for hospice care. HG died at her ICF MR with her family and personal care staff present, at the age of 59, after having Alzheimer's disease for approximately six years.

Our Research Findings: The simple description of prevalence of dementia among our patients with developmental disabilities was 6% and for the comparison group the prevalence of dementia was 1%. In our study group of 54 individuals with autism there were no cases of dementia; this is probably due to the earlier age at entry into the study. In fact the age at entry was 26 years for those with autism compared to 34 years for those with Down syndrome and 40 years for the comparison patients.

Thus, with less than 10 years of follow-up time the patients with autism simply did not develop dementia during the window of observation. The group with the highest prevalence was the adults with Down syndrome, with a prevalence of 19 percent.

We have data on age, the one well established risk factor for the development of dementia. For each year of age the risk for dementia increased 13% (Adjusted Odds Ratio 1.13, 95% Confidence Interval 1.10-1.16, p<0.001). Diabetes was also a statistically significant risk factor for dementia (Adjusted Odds Ratio 2.94, 95% Confidence Interval 1.47-5.86, p=0.002). Having a lower BMI was associated with lower risk for dementia (Adjusted Odds Ratio 0.93, 95% Confidence Interval 0.88-0.98, p=0.011).

When these confounders were in the predictive logistic regression models the adjusted odds ratio (and 95% confidence interval) was statistically significantly higher for all of the developmental disability groups, expect autism since there were no cases of dementia in this group. For those with CP the risk was 5 fold, for those with MR with or without a psychiatric diagnosis the risk was 6-7 fold higher compared to the comparison group. As expected the risk for the group with Down syndrome was extremely high (Adjusted Odds Ratio 67) for having dementia. The odds ratio, after controlling for confounders, for each of the DD groups are shown in Table 2.

We also used survival analysis to look at the hazard ratio for onset of dementia for the study participants who did not have it when they entered care at the two practices. As expected the results were very similar to the logistic regression results. The hazard ratio was the highest for those with Down syndrome, followed by those with MR. The hazard ratio for those with cerebral palsy was not significant and there were no new cases of dementia for those with autism (Table 3).

Implications from our study findings: The high risk for developing dementia for adults with cerebral palsy, Down syndrome, and mental retardation with and without mental illness, needs to make physicians alert for the identification of the symptoms. The odds ratios for prevalence of dementia were extremely high (Adjusted OR 67) for the group with Down syndrome. We hope these results prompt medical practices to do regular mental status screenings, followed by diagnostic testing, for adults with developmental disabilities as well as other high risk groups.

Providers need to be alert to changes in mental status in all adults with developmental disabilities, not just those with Down syndrome. Medical intervention can be tried following early diagnosis, and families and agencies can receive guidance as they anticipate the need for intensified caregiving arrangements. Families and agencies need to be prepared to provide more care as people survive into old age with developmental disabilities.

Table 1. Prevalence of dementia for adults with no disability and by developmental disability group for known risk factors

prevalence (ever)	without disability	All DD	Autism	Down syndrome	Cerebral Palsy	MR with Psychiatric Illness	MR
All	1809	694	54	58	163	152	267
	1.2	6.3	0.0	19.0	3.1	7.2	6.4
Gender							
Male	0.8	7.3	0.0	14.7	2.7	8.1	9.7
Female	1.5	5.2	0.0	25.0	3.4	6.4	2.5
Race							
White	1.3	6.5	0.0	14.0	3.8	9.3	6.5
African American	1.1	6.3	0.0	35.7	1.8	5.2	6.4
Other	0.0	0.0	0.0	0.0	0.0	0.0	0.0
Severity of Primary Disability							
Mild	n/a	n/a	0.0	16.7	4.0	6.7	7.1
Moderate	n/a	n/a	0.0	12.5	1.8	9.5	5.0
Severe	n/a	n/a	0.0	20.5	3.5	7.3	6.4
Residential Type							
Least Restrictive Environment	n/a	4.5	0.0	16.7	0.0	0.0	5.6
Most Restrictive Environment	n/a	3.9	0.0	18.8	1.7	2.8	3.8

Table 2. Logistic Regression Adjusted* Odds Ratio for developing Dementia, by developmental disability group

Groups	N	Prevalence	Adjusted* Odds Ratio	Lower Confidence Interval	Upper Confidence Interval	P-Value
Comparison	1809	1.2	1.00			
Autism	54	0.0				
Cerebral Palsy	163	19.0	**5.09**	**1.64**	**15.76**	**0.005**
Down syndrome	58	3.1	**66.62**	**25.00**	**177.57**	**0.001**
MR with Psychiatric Illness	152	7.2	**7.59**	**2.97**	**19.38**	**0.001**
MR Only	267	6.4	**8.69**	**4.11**	**18.36**	**0.001**

* controlling for medical site, age, race, gender, tobacco use, diabetes, BMI.
Bold indicates statistically significantly different from the comparison group.

Table 3. Adjusted* Hazard Ratio for development of dementia for each developmental disability group

Groups	n	Hazard Ratio	P-Value
Comparison	1809		
Autism	54		
Cerebral Palsy	161	2.13	0.124
Down syndrome	58	**34.73**	**0.001**
MR with Psychiatric Illness	151	**4.51**	**0.001**
MR Only	262	**4.73**	**0.001**

* adjusted for medical site, age, race, gender, BMI, diabetes, tobacco use.
Bold indicates statistically significantly different from the comparison group.

Implications for Case Study: The rapid decline of a high functioning individual like HG demonstrates the importance of both medical intervention and community supports. In this case the medical interventions failed but the family and support staff continued to intensify the care they provided during the last six years of HG's life. A team approach to care is needed when individuals with DD develop dementia since the manifestations are hard for families and staff to cope with and the popular press suggests medical interventions can produce dramatic results. Tracking and reporting frequency and intensity of behaviors are important in a condition that is characterized by decline. In the case of HG the medical interventions failed but the family physician continued to provide regular follow-up and supportive care. In addition Dr. P's longstanding relationship with HG, her family, and support staff, allowed him to know when hospice services should be provided, again providing an increased level of support for HG.

References

Bird, TD, Miller BL. Chapter 350: Alzheimer's Disease and Other Dementias. In *Harrison's Internal Medicine,* Internet access June 1, 2007, http://www.accessmedicine.com. proxy.med.sc.edu

Boustani M, Peterson B, Hanson L, Harris R, Lohr KN. Screening for Dementia in Primary Care: A Summary of the Evidence for the U.S. Preventive Services Task Force. *Ann. Intern. Med.*, 2003 138, 927-37.

Cooper B, Bickel H, Schaufele M. Early development and progression of dementing illness in the elderly: a general-practice based study. *Psycholog. Med.*, 1996 26, 411-19.

Evans DA, Funkenstein HH, Albert MS, Scherr PA, Cook NR, Chown MJ, et al. Prevalence of Alzheimer's disease in a community population of older persons. Higher than previously reported. *JAMA*, 1989 262, 2551-6.

Evans DA, Smith LA, Scherr PA, Albert MS, Funkenstein HH, Hebert LE. Risk of death from Alzheimer's disease in a community population of older persons. *Am. J. Epidemiol*, 1991 134, 403-12.

Janicki MP, Heller T, Seltzer GB, Hogg J. Practice guidelines for the clinical assessment and care management of Alzheimer's disease and other dementias among adults with intellectual disability. *Journal of Intellectual Disability Research*, 1996, 40, 374-382.

Janicki MP, Dalton AJ. Dementia and public policy considerations. In: M.P. Janicki and A.J. Dalton (Eds.). *Dementia, aging, and intellectual disabilities: A handbook.* Philadelphia PA: Taylor and Francis; 1999; 388-414.

Janicki MP, Dalton AJ. Prevalence of Dementia and Impact on Intellectual Disability Services. *Ment. Retard.*, 2000 38, 276-288.

Lai F, Williams RS. A prospective study of Alzheimer disease in Down syndrome. *Archives of Neurology*, 1989 46, 849-853.

Lagaay A, van der Meij J, Hijmans W. Validation of medical history taking as part of a population based survey in subjects aged 85 and over. *Br. Med. J.,* 1992 304, 1091-92.

McDowell I, Hill G, Lindsay J, Helliwell B, et al. Canadian study of health and aging: study methods and prevalence of dementia. *CMAJ,* 1994 150, 899-913.

Med Track Alert. View a condition, Alzheimer's disease [online]. 2007, March 20. Available from: http://www.medtrackalert.com/ViewCondition.asp?id=269:

O'Connor D, Pollitt P, Hyde J, Brook C, Reiss B, Roth M. Do general practitioners miss dementia in elderly patients? *Br. Med. J.*, 1988 297, 1107-10.

Olafsdottir M, Skoog I, Marcusson J. Detection of dementia in primary care: the Linkoping study. *Dement. Geriatr. Cogn. Disord.*, 2000 11, 223-29.

Patterson CJ, Gauthier S, Bergman H, Cohen CA, Feightner JW, Feldman H, et al. The recognition, assessment and management of dementing disorders: conclusions from the Canadian Consensus Conference on Dementia. *CMAJ,* 1999 160, S1-15.

U.S. General Accounting Office. Alzheimer's Disease: Estimates of prevalence in the United States. Washington, DC: U.S. General Accounting Office; 1998. Publication HEHS 98-16.

U.S. Office of Technology Assessment. Losing a million minds: confronting the tragedy of AD and other dementias. Washington, DC: US Government Printing Office; 1987.

Valcour V, Masaki K, Curb J, Blanchette P. The detection of dementia in the primary care setting. *Arch. Intern. Med.*, 2000 160, 2964-68.

Visser FE, Aldenkamp AP, van Huffelen AC, Kuilman M, Overweg J, van Wijk J. Prospective study of the prevalence of Alzheimer-type dementia in institutionalized individuals with Down syndrome. *Am. J. Ment. Retard.*, 1997 101, 400-412.

Wherett J. Neurological aspects. In: M.P. Janicki and A.J. Dalton (Eds.). *Dementia, aging, and intellectual disabilities: A handbook.* Philadelphia, PA: Taylor and Francis; 1999; 90-102.

Zigman WB, Schupf N, Zigman A, Silverman W. Aging and Alzheimer disease in people with mental retardation. *International Review of Research in Mental Retardation*, 1993 19, 41-70.

Chapter X

Asthma

The Research Questions: What is the prevalence of asthma among adults with developmental disabilities and how does this compare to other adults, after controlling for demographic characteristics? For those adults who do not have asthma when they enter the family medicine practice sites under study, are there differences in the incidence of asthma among the impairment groups compared to those without a disability?

Definition of Asthma and Prevalence in the General Population: Asthma is characterized by intermittent airway obstruction, bronchial smooth muscle cell hyper-reactivity to broncho-constrictors, and chronic bronchial inflammation. The etiology of asthma is heterogeneous with a number of established risk factors (Renauld et al, 2001).

The National Health Interview Survey (NHIS), a population-based survey of U.S households from the mid 1990s, estimated that 5.5% of U.S. residents (approximately 14.5 million people), have asthma (Adams, Hendershot, and Marano et al, 1999). By 2005, the lifetime prevalence in persons over the age of 18 years and older was 11% and 7% reported currently having the conditions. The age-adjusted percentage of asthma was 12.6% for females, 8.7% for males and 8.31% for African-American and 7.1% in whites. Prevalence estimates were based on a positive response to the question, "During the past 12 months, did you have asthma?" (Pleis and Lethbridge-Cejku et al, 2006)

The prevalence of asthma has been increasing in all age and racial groups during the past two decades. The variation in prevalence rates for racial and ethnic groups probably results from differences in genetic, environmental, social, and cultural influences (Coultas, Gong, and Grad et al, 1994). Factors affecting increased asthma prevalence include obesity and exposure to environmental irritants. The population has become increasingly sedentary, spending more time indoors where the exposure to allergens, such as mold, dust mites, and cockroach dust, is more prevalent. In addition, the increased prevalence of allergic rhinitis and atopy related to exposure to allergens at an early age is associated with the prevalence of asthma.

State prevalence estimates of asthma are provided by the Behavioral Risk Factor Surveillance System (BRFSS). The 2002 report of adult self-reported current asthma prevalence for South Carolina was 5.8% (standard error 0.51) with a 95% confidence interval of 4.9-6.8 (Centers for Disease Control and Prevention et al, 2004).

Literature Review of asthma in adults with Developmental Disability: There is little in the literature about the risk for asthma among adults with developmental disabilities. In a longitudinal cohort study of 1453 people with Down syndrome and 460,000 people without disabilities, the Relative Risk for asthma among those with Down syndrome was statistically significantly reduced (RR 0.4, 95% Confidence Interval 0.2-0.6) (Goldacre, Wotton, Seagroatt, and Yeates et al, 2004). There are no specific studies of asthma in people with other types of developmental disabilities although asthma has been included in some surveys of health conditions.

What is the Conceptual Framework for this question?: The prevalence of asthma is increasing and the population subgroups with the largest increase are minority children and adults who live in poverty. People with developmental disability have high rates of poverty and many grew up in impoverished conditions, however it has not been established if this group has a high prevalence of asthma.

For those with both developmental disability and asthma there is a substantial challenge related to self-management of the symptoms of asthma. Having a working knowledge of the disease process is needed to maximize disease-management and the information is both complex and abstract, therefore it poses a substantial challenge for people with developmental disabilities, who struggle with cognitive tasks. Physicians and nurses need to discuss asthma action plans with their patients with developmental disabilities and encourage the use of tools and personal supports to help patients achieve better control of their disease.

Case Study: SD is a 55 year old, African American female with mild mental retardation (ICD9 317), as well as persistent, chronic asthma (ICD9 493.00). In addition, she has bi-lateral hearing loss (ICD9 389.9) and seizure disorder (ICD9 345.10) controlled by phenytoin (Dilantin). SD was originally living in a community apartment setting and working part time in the kitchen for a disability agency workshop, and part time in a large community residential facility for patients with developmental disabilities. SD has been under the care of Dr. T. at the University affiliated family medicine center. She has life long asthma and a history of multiple hospitalizations related to exacerbations of the condition.

On two occasions in the past three years she required admission to the intensive care unit and at this time Dr. T. transferred her care to a pulmonologist, Dr. M. Following hospital discharge SD was tried on a multitude of regimens, however in part due to the fact that she lived alone, she did not have the supports to get the acute respiratory care she needs on a regular basis. SD needed to confer with someone when her breathing started to become difficult. She also needed to use the prescribed combination of medications, based on the presenting symptoms, and she had to arrange transportation to the doctor's office or emergency room, on an as needed basis. After her last hospitalization one year ago, SD moved to a CTH II (community treatment home) where staff and transportation are available 24 hours a day.

Since moving to the CTH II SD has done well using an ipratropium bromide and albuterol sulfate aerosol (Combivent), Fluticasone inhaler, and albuterol (Proventil) on an as needed basis. Dr. T. received written consults from Dr. M. on a regular basis and sees SD twice a year. With the supervision of Dr. T. and the support staff at the CTH, SD continues on a long acting beta agent as well as the other medications. She is now stabilized on this regimen for about one year without a re-hospitalization. SD is seen every 2-3 months in the family medicine office and she still has mild expiratory wheezing and evidence of restrictive changes on her spirometry. SD sees Dr. M. bi-annually and her pulmonary function tests have remained stable. SD continues to work in the kitchen at the community workshop and is involved in a number of community activities.

Our Research Findings: In our study the case definition of asthma required both of the following: *1*) physician diagnosis that the individual has asthma and *2*) reported prescription of an asthma medication since diagnosis. These medications include: inhaled steroids, oral or intravenous steroids, theophylline, anhydrous (Uniphyl) , cromolyn sodium aerosol (Intal) or nedocromil, leukotriene modifiers, albterol (Proventil), fluticasone propionate, and salmeterol (Advair). To meet our case definition participants had to fulfill both criteria in the past year.

Table 1 shows the prevalence of asthma for each study group by the characteristics of the group. Overall the two groups with the highest asthma prevalence were those with both mental retardation and a psychiatric illness (6.6%) and those with no disability (6.1%). The group with the lowest overall prevalence was those with autism (1.9%). These rates reflect one characteristic at a time and do not take into account the other factors.

We used logistic regression analysis to calculate the adjusted odds ratios for each of the developmental disability groups compared to the patients without disabilities with adjusting for all of the risk factors. We evaluated the association of all the risk factors with asthma prevalence and found age (Adjusted Odds Ratio 0.98; 95% Confidence Interval 0.97-1.00; p=0.013) and BMI (Adjusted Odds Ratio 1.03; 95% Confidence Interval 1.0-1.05; p=0.04) were statistically significantly associated with the odds of having asthma. Then when we analyzed the risk for asthma for each of the developmental disability groups compared to the comparison group, after adjusting for age, race, gender, BMI, diabetes, and tobacco use, none of the DD sub-groups had statistically significantly increased odds for asthma (Table 2).

Finally, we used survival analysis to compare the hazard function for the onset of asthma for the members of each disability group who entered the study without asthma compared to the comparison group who entered the study without asthma. Again, we explored the co-variates of age, race, gender, BMI, diabetes and smoking and found they were statistically significantly associated with the onset of asthma. We controlled for each of these variables in the Cox-proportional Hazard models which are show in Table 3. There was no significant association with asthma for any of the developmental disability sub-groups when compared to the patients without disabilities.

Implications from our study findings: We found that neither the prevalence nor incidence of asthma was statistically significantly different for the subgroups with developmental disabilities compared to the adults without disabilities. This is observed in the Southern US where the study was conducted and the rates of asthma are usually reported to be higher than the 5.5% estimate for the US population. In our comparison group the prevalence of asthma was 6.1% and there was no statistically significant difference in the prevalence or incidence in the adults with DD.

Implications for Case Study: The management of asthma in patients with developmental disabilities is complicated by the need to minimize triggers for exacerbations and make timely decisions about escalating symptoms. Adults with developmental disabilities are more likely to be poorer than the general population, so they often live in substandard housing where many of the exacerbating triggers for asthma are present. The challenge of self-management of asthma for adults with developmental disabilities are confounded by the inherent limitations in abstract thinking and problem solving skills that are associated with the primary disability. This is especially difficult when the individual with DD lives alone or without sufficient supports to determine if an emergency is developing. SD improved her asthma management after moving to a group home where these supports were readily available. Nonetheless, management of SD's asthma was facilitated by her close relationship with her primary care physician and pulmonologist who was able to manage her condition with the knowledge of her functional status and her living situation.

Table 1. Prevalence of asthma by adults with no disability and developmental disability group, by known risk factors

prevalence (ever)	No disability	All DD	Autism	Down syndrome	Cerebral Palsy	MR with Psychiatric Illness	MR
All	1809	694	54	58	163	152	267
	6.1	4.2	1.9	3.5	4.3	6.6	3.4
Gender							
Male	6.1	4.3	2.4	5.9	6.8	4.1	3.5
Female	6.2	4.0	0.0	0.0	2.3	9.0	3.3
Race							
White	6.4	4.1	2.6	2.3	2.8	8.0	3.9
African American	6.2	4.4	0.0	7.1	7.1	5.2	2.7
Other	2.4	0.0	0.0	0.0	0.0	0.0	0.0
Severity of primary disability							
Mild	n/a	n/a	0.0	0.0	4.0	7.8	5.1
Moderate	n/a	n/a	2.6	0.0	5.4	14.3	5.0
Severe	n/a	n/a	0.0	4.6	3.5	0.0	0.9
Residential Type							
Least Restrictive Environment	n/a	8.9	0.0	8.3	10.0	17.4	5.6
Most Restrictive Environment	n/a	3.9	0.0	0.0	6.9	2.8	3.8

Table 2. Logistic Regression adjusted* odds ratio for developing asthma among the developmental disability groups

Groups	n	Prevalence	Adjusted* Odds Ratio	Lower Confidence Interval	Upper Confidence Interval	P-Value
Comparison	1809	6.1	1.00			
Autism	54	1.9	0.28	0.04	2.10	0.217
Cerebral Palsy	163	3.5	0.87	0.38	1.97	0.736
Down syndrome	58	4.3	0.59	0.14	2.48	0.470
MR with Psychiatric Illness	152	6.6	1.12	0.55	2.28	0.760
MR Only	267	3.4	0.58	0.29	1.17	0.130

*adjusting for medical site, age, race, gender, BMI, diabetes, and smoking.

Table 3. Survival Analysis, hazard * for onset of asthma, by developmental disability group

Groups	N	Hazard Ratio	P-Value
Comparison	1790		
Autism	54	0.62	0.633
Cerebral Palsy	162	1.12	0.752
Down syndrome	58	0.63	0.521
MR with Psychiatric Illness	151	1.06	0.863
MR Only	261	0.63	0.182

* adjusted for medical site, race, gender, age, BMI, tobacco use.

References

Adams PF, Hendershot GE, Marano MA. Current estimates from the National Health Interview Survey, 1996. *Vital Health Stat.* 10, 1999 200, 1-203.

Centers for Disease Control and Prevention. Asthma prevalence and control characteristics by race/ethnicity –United States, 2002. *MMWR*, 2004 53, 145-148.

Coultas DB, Gong H, Grad R, Handler A, McCurdy SA, Player R, Rhoades ER, Samet SM, Thomas A, Westley M. *Respiratory diseases in minorities of the United States*, 1994 149, S93-131.

Goldacre MJ, Wotton CJ, Seagroatt V, Yeates D. Cancers and immune related diseases associated with Down's syndrome: a record linkage study. *Arch. Dis. Child,* 2004 89, 1014-1017.

Pleis JR, Lethbridge-Cejku M. Summary health statistics for U.S. adults: National Health Interview Survey, 2005. *Vital Health Stat.* 10, 2006 232, 1-153.

Renauld JC. New insights into the role of cytokines in asthma. *J. Clin. Pathol.,* 2001 54, 577-89.

Chapter XI

Chronic Obstructive Pulmonary Disease

The Research Questions: What is the prevalence of chronic obstructive pulmonary disease (COPD) among adults with developmental disabilities and how does this compare to other adults, after controlling for risk characteristics? For those adults who do not have chronic obstructive pulmonary disease when they enter the family medicine practice sites under study, are there differences in the incidence of COPD among the impairment groups compared to those without a disability?

Definition of Chronic Obstructive Pulmonary Disease (COPD) and Prevalence of COPD in the General Population: Chronic obstructive pulmonary disease (COPD) is characterized by the progressive development of airflow limitation that is not fully reversible (American Thoracic Society et al, 1995). The term COPD encompasses chronic obstructive bronchitis, with obstruction of small airways, and emphysema, with enlargement of air spaces and destruction of lung parenchyma, loss of lung elasticity, and closure of small airways (Petty et al, 2000).The most substantial risk factor for the development of COPD is tobacco smoking. It has been established that inflammation plays a key role in chronic obstructive pulmonary disease (Rona et al, 2004).

COPD is rarely diagnosed before age 35 years, and approximately 45% of those with the diagnosis have an asthmatic component (American Thoracic Society et al, 1995). In the third U.S. National Health and Nutrition Examination Survey, airflow obstruction was found in approximately 14% of white male smokers, as compared with approximately 3% of white male nonsmokers (Pauwels, 2001). COPD is now the fourth leading cause of death in the United States, and it is the only common cause of death that is increasing in incidence. The importance of COPD as a cause of death is possibly underestimated, since COPD can contribute to other common causes of death, including heart disease and cancer (Barnes, et al, 2000).

Chronic obstructive pulmonary disease (COPD) is the most common chronic lung disease seen in the offices of primary care clinicians. In the United States, COPD is the fourth leading cause of death behind coronary heart disease, cancer, and stroke, and accounts for more than $30 billion in annual health care costs (National Heart, Lung, and Blood

Association et al, 2003). An estimated 16 million adults are affected by COPD, and each year 120,000 Americans die of the disease (Mannino, Homa, and Akinbami et al, 2002).

Results of the 2001 National Health Interview Survey indicate that approximately 16 million adults aged 18 years of age and older have received a COPD diagnosis from a physician (National Heart, Lung, and Blood Institute et al, 2003; COPD International Website et al, 2007). And the Third National Health and Nutrition Examination Survey (NHANES III) found that greater than 70% of 16,000 surveyed US adults who had abnormal lung function (measured by spirometry) characteristic of COPD had not been diagnosed with COPD (Petty et al, 2000). It is likely, therefore, that the prevalence of COPD is underestimated and is closer to 40 to 50 million (National Heart, Lung, and Blood Institute et al, 2003).

The major risk factor for the development of COPD is the inhalation of tobacco smoke and some chemicals (Pauwels, Buist, and Calverley et al, 2001). Smoking (including cigarettes, pipes, and cigars) is the cause of approximately 85% to 90% of COPD cases (Kornmann, Beeh, and Beier et al, 2003). Research indicates between 70% to 90% of smokers develop COPD, and 20% of these patients develop the disease rapidly (American Lung Association, et al 2006).

Literature Review of COPD in Adults with Developmental Disability: Like asthma, there are no published studies that specifically focus on COPD among adults with developmental disabilities.

What is the Conceptual Framework for this question?: The onset of Chronic Obstructive Pulmonary Disease (COPD) is primary related to cigarette smoking (Pauwels, Buist, and Calverley et al, 2001). Smoking (including cigarettes, pipes, and cigars) is the cause of 85% to 90% of COPD cases (Kornmann, Beeh, Beier et al, 2003), however because many smokers with mild to moderate symptoms are not currently diagnosed with COPD the prevalence estimates in the general population are probably underestimating the problem. A small percentage of smokers do not appear to develop clinically significant COPD, suggesting that genetic factors may modify the risk of developing disease in this small group.

The issues related to identifying the prevalence of COPD in adults with developmental disabilities are two fold. First we need to establish an estimate of smoking in this group, in order to know who is at risk. Second we need to be confident about the diagnosis of the condition. In this study we were able to record smoking status on the patient's medical record for all the individuals in the case and comparison group. This information was recorded by physicians and nurses, prompted by a question in the electronic medical record, but as in all secondary data about smoking data, the physician or nurse is only able to record smoking if the patient or the caregiver acknowledges the behavior. The adults with DD often are accompanied to their medical visit by a caregiver and this individual is more likely to report smoking, if it is occurring. Thus, we expect to have underestimated the prevalence of smoking, especially in the comparison group.

In reference to the second issue of under-diagnosis of COPD among individuals with mild to moderate symptoms, we again expect this is more problematic for the comparison group who might be more inclined to under report since the adults with DD often are accompanied to their medical visit by a caregiver and this individual is more likely to provide an objective assessment of the problem. Thus, we need to interpret our finding about the prevalence of COPD among smokers in the DD and comparison group.

Case Study: KC is a 54 year old male with mild mental retardation (IDC9 317) and a 3 pack a day cigarette smoking habit that he has maintained for over 20 years. KC has been under the care of Dr. M. for over ten years and they have discussed the implications of smoking at most of the early visits when Dr. M. felt it was imperative to get KC into a smoking cessation program. KC has consistently refused the referral to a smoking based program in the medical practice and Dr. M. continued to ask about his smoking habit at every visit. KC has had 2 hospitalizations for pneumonia; the most recent being three months ago. Since his first hospitalization KC has been under the care of a pulmonologist who sees him every 3 months. His situation is complicated by a very inactive lifestyle – he refuses to participate in workshop or take part in other physical or work activity. In addition he has hyperlipidemia requiring medication and KC refuses to follow a lower cholesterol diet. He has gained weight over the past ten years and his BMI is now 32. Pulmonary function tests confirm moderate obstructive pulmonary disease with a mild restrictive component (ICD9 496) and he requires steroid inhaler twice a day as well as a combination inhaler with brand of albuterol, USP Inhalation Aerosol (Proventil), ipratropium bromide, and albuterol sulfate Inhalation Aerosol (Combivent) four times per day.

In addition to his two hospitalizations for pneumonia, KC has had multiple episodes of bronchitis the past several years. Dr. M. has offered immunizations at all his visits but KC refuses yearly flu shots and pneumococcal vaccine polyvalent (Pneumovax). KC wants few supports in his daily life and he only agrees to infrequent contact with his disability service coordinator. Dr. M. has talked to the service coordinator on numerous occasions and both are concerned that KC's strong will has complicated his treatment. He understands instructions and the arguments for stopping smoking and getting immunized against pneumonia and influenza, yet he continues to refuse to consider even cutting down on his smoking or getting the immunizations. At the present time KC's family is trying to persuade him to move to move to a more restrictive environment since his COPD and associated acute respiratory illnesses need more surveillance and better management.

Our Research Findings: In our study the case definition of chronic obstructive pulmonary disease required both of the following: 1) physician diagnosis that the individual has COPD and 2) prescription of COPD medications since diagnosis. These medications include: inhaled steroids, oral or intravenous steroids, theophylline , anhydrous (Uniphyl), cromolyn sodium inhalation aerosol (Intal), ipratropium bromide, and albuterol sulfate (Combivent, Proventil), Nedocromil, leukotriene modifiers, and salmeterol (Advair).

In our dataset 20.1% of current smokers have COPD, 17.7% of past smokers have COPD, and 1.7% of non-smokers have COPD. We also observed 17.4% of the adults with developmental disabilities are current smokers, 4.8% are past smokers, and 77.8% never smoked. Finally, 29.9% of the adults without disabilities are current smokers, 13.8% are past smokers, and 56.3% never smoked.

Table 1 shows the prevalence of COPD for each study group by the characteristics of the group.

Overall the two groups with the highest COPD prevalence were those with mental retardation and a psychiatric illness (10.5%). Adults with no disability had COPD prevalence of (9.1%). The group with the lowest overall prevalence was those with Down syndrome (1.7%) and autism (1.9%). It is also noteworthy that males were more likely to have COPD than females, and whites were more likely to have COPD than African-Americans. These rates reflect one characteristic at a time and do not take into account the other factors.

We used logistic regression analysis to calculate the adjusted odds ratios for COPD for each of the developmental disability groups compared to the patients without disabilities, after adjusting for all of the risk factors. However, first we evaluated the association of a few important risk factors for COPD prevalence and found age was a statistically significant risk factor that increased the odds of having COPD (Adjusted Odds Ratio 1.06; 95% Confidence Interval 1.05-1.08; p=0.001). In addition race was a significant risk factor, being African Americans was significantly associated with being less likely to have COPD (Adjusted Odds Ratio 0.64; 95% Confidence Interval 0.45-0.91; p=0.012). Finally, the well-established risk factor of smoking was associated with a significantly elevated risk for having COPD (Adjusted Odds Ratio 18.53; 95% Confidence Interval 11.12-30.88; p=0.001). Then we analyzed the risk for COPD for each of the developmental disability groups compared to the comparison group, after adjusting for the risk factors (Table 2). Only the group with MR had statistically significantly increased odds for COPD; approximately two fold higher compared to the comparison group ((Adjusted Odds Ratio 1.96; 95% Confidence Interval 1.12-3.44), p=0.025).

We then stratified by smoking status to determine if there were group differences for people who never smoked compared to people who previously or currently smoke. The results in Table 3 show that those with autism, cerebral palsy and MR only had statistically significant reduced odds of having COPD, if they never smoked compared to the comparison group who never smoked.

Table 4 shows that for the people who previously or currently smoke there was no statistical difference in the odds of having COPD between each of the developmental disability groups and the comparison group.

Finally, using survival analysis we compared the hazard function for the onset of COPD for the members of each disability group who entered the study without COPD compared to the comparison group who entered the study without COPD (Table 5). There were three statistically significant risk factors for the development of COPD: being female had a protective effect (Hazard Ratio 0.72, p=0.033) and being younger also had a protective effect (Hazard Ratio 0.93, p=0.001). Again, as expected being a smoker was a risk factor (Hazard Ratio 6.01, p=0.001). There were no differences in the risk of onset of COPD between any of the groups with developmental disabilities compared to the adults with no disabilities.

Table 1. Prevalence of Chronic Obstructive Pulmonary Disease for those with no disability and each developmental disability group, by known risk factors

prevalence (ever)	No disability	All DD	Autism	Down syndrome	Cerebral Palsy	MR with Psychiatric Illness	MR
All	1809	694	54	58	163	152	267
	9.1	6.3	1.9	1.7	3.1	10.5	7.9
Gender							
Male	10.1	7.9	2.4	0.0	5.4	12.2	10.3
Female	8.4	4.6	0.0	4.2	1.1	9.0	4.9
Race							
White	11.4	7.5	2.6	2.3	4.7	13.3	9.2
African Americans	7.3	4.8	0.0	0.0	0.0	7.8	6.4
Other	4.9	0.0	0.0	0.0	0.0	0.0	0.0
Severity of Primary Disability							
Mild	n/a	n/a	0.0	0.0	6.0	13.3	12.2
Moderate	n/a	n/a	2.3	0.0	1.8	14.3	5.0
Severe	n/a	n/a	0.0	2.3	1.8	2.4	5.5
Residential Type							
Least Restrictive Environment	n/a	7.1	0.0	0.0	5.0	4.4	11.1
Most Restrictive Environment	n/a	3.4	0.0	0.0	3.5	5.6	3.8

Table 2. Logistic Regression, Adjusted Odds Ratio* for prevalence of Chronic Obstructive Pulmonary Disease, by developmental disability group

Groups	n	Prevalence	Adjusted Odds Ratio	Lower Confidence Interval	Upper Confidence Interval	P-Value
Comparison	1809	9.1	1.00			
Autism	54	1.9	1.34	0.14	13.08	0.802
Cerebral Palsy	163	1.7	1.59	0.56	4.52	0.387
Down syndrome	58	3.1	0.68	0.09	5.48	0.720
MR with Psychiatric Illness	152	10.5	1.71	0.91	3.12	0.096
MR Only	267	7.9	**1.96**	**1.12**	**3.44**	**0.025**

*adjusted for medical site, age, race, gender, and BMI.
Bold indicates statistically significantly different from the comparison group.

Table 3. Logistic Regression, Adjusted Odds Ratio* for prevalence of COPD among people who *never smoked*, by developmental disability group

Groups	n	Prevalence	Adjusted Odds Ratio	Lower Confidence Interval	Upper Confidence Interval	P-Value
Comparison	1019	1.9	1.00			
Autism	**52**	0.0	**0.20**	**0.05**	**0.83**	**0.0262**
Cerebral Palsy	**150**	**1.3**	**0.58**	**0.35**	**0.96**	**0.0334**
Down syndrome	52	1.9	0.49	0.21	1.19	0.1175
MR with Psychiatric Illness	91	3.3	1.13	0.67	1.91	0.6535
MR Only	**195**	**0.5**	**0.46**	**0.28**	**0.74**	**0.0013**

*adjusted for medical site, age, race, gender, and BMI.
Bold indicates statistically significantly different from the comparison group.

Table 4. Logistic Regression, Adjusted Odds Ratio* for prevalence of COPD among people who *ever smoked* (past and current), by developmental disability group

Groups	n	Prevalence	Adjusted Odds Ratio	Lower Confidence Interval	Upper Confidence Interval	P-Value
Comparison	790	18.5	1.00			0.9995
Autism	2	50.0				0.8286
Cerebral Palsy	13	21.3	1.16	0.31	4.33	0.8490
Down syndrome	6	0.0				0.3488
MR with Psychiatric Illness	61	21.3	1.33	0.73	2.43	0.2726
MR Only	72	27.8	1.37	0.78	2.39	

*adjusted for medical site, age, race, gender, and BMI.

Table 5. Survival Analysis, adjusted hazard rate* for onset of chronic obstructive pulmonary disease, by developmental disability group

Groups	n	Hazard Ratio	P-Value
Comparison	1796		
Autism	54	1.12	0.910
Cerebral Palsy	162	0.80	0.625
Down syndrome	58	0.45	0.428
MR with Psychiatric Illness	152	1.15	0.613
MR Only	262	1.11	0.683

*adjusted for medical site, race, gender, BMI, diabetes and tobacco use.

Implications from our study findings: The results of our study indicate people with MR were at significantly higher risk for having COPD. This needs to be understood in light of the finding that the risk of developing COPD for the group with MR who entered the practice without it was not statistically significantly elevated. Overall approximately 18 percent of the adults with MR were smokers and it is important that physicians to remember to counsel these patients, as well as all others, for smoking cessation. In this study the prevalence of COPD was higher among the patients with MR but the incidence was not significantly different from the comparison group. Thus we can assume that some people with MR entered the practice with COPD already established. Table 1 shows us that for the group with MR the risk groups were males, who are white, with mild MR and living in the least restrictive environment.

Implications for Case Study: COPD is highly associated with smoking and physicians need to counsel patients with MR to abstain from smoking and quit smoking if they have already begun when they enter the medical practice. Most smoking cessation programs can readily accommodate an individual with mild MR, but this is not the case for adults with moderate to severe levels of function. In all cases the use of medicines to reduce tobacco cravings should be considered, but this would require there are sufficient family or caregiver supports to assure appropriate use of the medications.

Although vaccine prophylaxis is important to consider for all adults, once COPD is established, it is especially important to offer both influenza and pneumovax immunization to prevent exacerbations. And since care for established COPD requires use of a substantial number of medications and medical regimes, it is important to have adequate supports for individuals with developmental disabilities and COPD.

References

American Lung Association. Chronic Obstructive Pulmonary Disease (COPD) *Fact Sheet.* August 2006.

American Thoracic Society. Standards for the diagnosis and care of patients with chronic obstructive pulmonary disease. *Am. J. Respir. Crit. Care Med,* 1995 152, S77-121.

Barnes PJ. Chronic obstructive pulmonary disease. *N. Engl. J. Med.,* 2000 343, 269–80.

Barr RG, Herbstman J, Speizer FE, Camargo CA. Validation on self-reported Chronic Obstructive Pulmonary disease in a cohort study of nurses. *Am. J. Epidemiol.,* 2002 155, 965-971.

Centers for Disease Control and Prevention. Current estimates from the National Health Interview Survey, 1995. Vital and health statistics. *MMWR,* 1995 444, 98-1527.

COPD International Web site. 2007 April 12. Available from: http://www.copd-international.com.

Coultas DB, Mapel D, Gagnon R, Lydick E. The health impact of undiagnosed airflow obstruction in a national sample of United States adults. *Am. J. Respir. Crit. Care Med,* 2001 164, 372-7.

Kornmann O, Beeh KM, Beier J. Newly diagnosed chronic obstructive pulmonary disease. Clinical features and distribution of the novel stages of Global Initiative for Obstructive Lung Disease. *Respiration,* 2003 70, 67-75.

Mannino DM, Ford ES, Redd SC: Obstructive and restrictive lung disease and markers of inflammation: data from the Third National Health and Nutrition Examination. *Am. J. Med.* 114:758–762, 2003.

Mannino D, Homa D, Akinbami LJ. Chronic obstructive pulmonary disease surveillance-- United States, 1971-2000. *MMWR,* 2002 51, 1-16.

National Heart, Lung, and Blood Institute. Chronic Obstructive Pulmonary Disease (COPD) *Data Fact Sheet.* March 2003.

Petty TL. Scope of the COPD problem in North America: early studies of prevalence and NHANES III data: basis for early identification and intervention. *Chest,* 2000 117, 326S-31S.

Pauwels RA, Buist AS, Calverley PM, et al. Global strategy for the diagnosis, management and prevention of chronic obstructive pulmonary disease. NHLBI/WHO Global Initiative for Chronic Obstructive Lung Disease (GOLD) Workshop Summary. *Am. J. Respir. Crit. Care Med.,* 2001 163, 1256-76.

Rona JS, Mittleman MA, Sheikh J, Hu FB, Manson JE, Colditz GA, Speizer FE, Barr RG, Camargo CA, Chronic obstructive pulmonary disease, asthma, and risk of type 2 diabetes in women. *Diabetes Care* 27, 2478-84, 2004.

Chapter XII

Epilepsy

The Research Questions: What is the prevalence of epilepsy among adults with developmental disabilities and how does this compare to other adults, after controlling for risk characteristics? For those adults who do not have epilepsy when they enter the family medicine practice sites under study, are there differences in the incidence of epilepsy among the subgroups with developmental disability, compared to those without a disability?

Definition of Epilepsy and Prevalence in the General Population: Epilepsy is a brain disorder in which clusters of neurons in the brain sometimes signal abnormally causing strange sensations, emotions, and behavior or seizures, muscle spasms, and loss of consciousness. A seizure is defined as a behavioral, motor, sensory, or cognitive event that is due to abnormal neuronal activity characterized by excessive hyper-synchronous neuronal discharges. Epilepsy is defined as recurrent seizures secondary to central nervous system dysfunction (NINDS, 2007).

It has been reported that 4-10% of children experience a seizure at some time in their lives. By age 20 however, only one percent of the general population has a diagnosis of seizures or epilepsy (Hauser et al, 1994). The distinction between seizures and epilepsy is based on number of events, with seizure being a single event and epilepsy a description of recurrent episodes.

Literature Review of Epilepsy in Adults with Developmental Disability: The literature on the prevalence of seizures and epilepsy among adults with developmental disabilities often relies on data from specialty settings, institutions, and registries. In these settings investigators have studied the co-morbidity of epilepsy associated with numerous childhood onset conditions including cerebral palsy (CP), autism, Down syndrome, and mental retardation (MR) (Brodtkrob et al, 2004; Johannsen and Christensen et al, 1996; Volkmar and Nelson et al, 1990).

Recent reports about children with CP indicate 35% have a history of epilepsy, with the highest prevalence in children with spastic hemiplegia (66%), followed by those with quadriplegia (43%), and diplegia (16%) (Singhi, Jagirdar, Khandelwal, and Malhi et al, 2003).

The prevalence of epilepsy in children with autism is estimated to be 5-38%, with age, cognitive level, and type of language disorder having the greatest predictive power (Acardi et al, 1994; Deykin and MacMahon et al, 1979; Mouridsen, Rich, and Isager et al, 1999; Tuchman and Rapin et al, 2002; Vokmar and Nelson et al, 1990).

The prevalence of epilepsy in Down syndrome has been reported to be 8-9% with a bimodal distribution, 40% starting with seizure activity before the age of one year and another 40% starting seizures during the period 20 to 30 years of age (Pueschel, Louis, and McKnight et al, 1991). As is the case with autism, prevalence is age related, and the proportion of adults with Down syndrome over the age of 50 years is reported to be 46% (McVicker, Shanks, and McClelland et al, 1994). The age of onset of epilepsy for adults with Down syndrome is distinct from onset of epilepsy for other causes of mental retardation. The overall mean age of onset was 37 years in one study in the United Kingdom, with a bimodal distribution. The first mode was before age 20 and the second mode was in the fifth and sixth decade of life. This is important since research found late-onset epilepsy in Down syndrome is associated with Alzheimer's disease, and early onset epilepsy is associated with an absence of dementia (Puri, Ho, and Singh et al, 2001).

A review article indicated the prevalence of epilepsy in adults with mental retardation and other intellectual disabilities ranged from 18.3-44% (Bowley and Kerr et al, 2000). The most recent report indicates 16% of individuals with mental retardation have epilepsy (Morgan, Baxter, and Kerr et al, 2003). A systematic review and meta-analysis of the incidence of epilepsy reports the age group with the highest incidence was children under the age of 18 years followed by the group over 60 years (Kotsopoulos, van Merode, Kessels, de Krom, Knottnerus et al, 2002). Another recent published report found there was a decline in the relative risk of epilepsy among people with mental retardation compared to the general population, resulting from increased mortality among individuals with co-existing epilepsy and intellectual disability (Morgan, Baxter, and Kerr et al, 2003).

The use of medication to control seizures is central to the treatment of epilepsy. The issue of over-treatment of epilepsy patients has been documented, however in patients with complex neurological conditions such as CP and other developmental disabilities multi-drug treatment is often necessary (Deckers et al, 2002). Since behavioral challenges and psychiatric disorders are more prevalent in individuals with mental retardation and epilepsy, careful monitoring of medications is imperative (Devinsky et al, 2002).

What is the Conceptual Framework for this question?: The biologic basis for mental retardation has been at the center of the nature-nurture debate about human intelligence for decades. There is consensus that the proportions are approximately equal with some argument about what constitutes the factors related to both nature and nurture. Is fetal exposure to a sexually transmitted disease or alcohol nature or nurture? What causes genetic defects? Are their exposures that impact the maternal or paternal stem cells? Researchers around the world have wondered what proportion of mental retardation results from neonatal insults, such as infection and chemical exposure, and how much latitude remains in brain development after birth to improve inborn abilities. Some epidemiologists have suggested epilepsy is a marker for brain damage in-utero and when epilepsy or other neurologic signs are associated with developmental delay the "nature" theory is supported. The absence of epilepsy or neurologic signs would suggest "nurture". This study looked at the risk for epilepsy in adults with developmental delay and higher prevalence of epilepsy could be interpreted in light of the "nature-nurture" paradigm.

Case Study: LE is a 41 year old with severe mental retardation (ICD9 318.1) who has suffered from epilepsy (ICD9 345.1) since her early years. She has lived in an ICF/MR facility for approximately 20 years, under the medical care of Dr. V., who is the Medical Director for the disability agency administering the group homes. Dr. V. is a family medicine physician who works closely with a group of specialists in cardiology, neurology, psychiatry and other specialties. Over the years Dr. V. and Dr. M., the neurologist have prescribed multiple combinations of medications for LE. Many of these combinations sedated her so that at times LE would be sleeping 16 hours per day and be difficult to arouse. Dr. M. found LE to be a challenging patient, but the close working relationship with Dr. V., and frequent phone calls back and forth have been extremely helpful. LE's seizures have been of the grand mal type and she has had as many as 20 in a month. Over the years, LE usually needs to take at least 4 medications daily to control her seizures. This regimen keeps her seizures to 4-6 per month, which both Dr. M. and Dr. V., as well as the direct care and nursing staff, agree is an acceptable level. If the physicians attempt to more tightly control her seizures the medications overly sedates LE or she experiences the toxic side effects of the medications.

Following a particularly difficult period of seizure control seven years ago, a vagal nerve stimulator was implanted in hopes that this would make it easier to reduce the severity and abort some of LE's seizures. Dr. M., the neurologist, also hoped the vagal nerve stimulator would allow them to decrease some of LE's medications. In hindsight the stimulator did not decrease the frequency of seizures, but at least during LE's waking hours the magnitude of the episodes seems to be reduced.

With the advent of newer anti-seizure medications and the vagal nerve stimulator LE has better control of the seizures with less sedation than previously. Presently she is taking zonisamide (Zonegran), oxcarbazepine (Trileptal) and levetircetam (Keppra). With these medications and the vagal nerve stimulator, and follow-up by both Dr. M. and Dr. V., LE's seizures are adequately controlled and she is not experiencing substantial side effects at this time.

Our Research Findings: Epilepsy was identified in both progress notes, the problem list, and the ICD-9 code of 345 or 780.39 was listed (World Health Organization et al, 2000). The severity of epilepsy was determined by reviewing the medications prescribed and the number, frequency and type of seizures. Since the study subjects were established patients in the two primary care clinics, physicians had more than a history of epilepsy to make a diagnosis. Most patients had consultation notes from a neurologist, EEG reports, CAT scan and diagnostic studies (McDermott, Moran, Platt, Wood, Isaac, and Dasari et al, 2005). If the diagnosis of epilepsy was in doubt, in most cases the physicians were able to take patients off mono-therapy to determine if seizures were persistent. If there was no evidence of seizures in the months following withdrawal from medication, a note was written on the medical record stating the diagnosis of epilepsy was not applicable. This note was read by our coders and verified by the study physician. As a result, in our study individuals with a history of a single seizure or an acute event triggering the seizure, with no need for ongoing medication, were not identified as having epilepsy.

Two levels of epilepsy were used for coding: moderate and severe. If one or two drugs were required to control the epilepsy and there were few and infrequent break-through or partial seizures, the individual was considered a case with moderate epilepsy.

If the epilepsy activity required increasing doses and/or at least three medications, or use of medical device (e.g. vagal nerve stimulator) for control, the individual was coded as a case with severe epilepsy (McDermott, Moran, Platt, Wood, Isaac, and Dasari et al, 2005).

Table 1 shows the overall prevalence of epilepsy is substantially higher for all the developmental disability subgroups, ranging from 14% for adults with Down syndrome to 37% for CP, compared to the controls (1.0%). The vast majority of epilepsy cases were classified as moderate, responding to one or two medications to achieve control. The case group with the highest proportion of severe epilepsy was CP with MR, requiring three or more medications, a vagal nerve stimulator, or other medical device or surgery. It is noteworthy that there were no cases of severe epilepsy in the groups with Down syndrome or CP without MR. Only one case of severe epilepsy was identified in the group with autism. However, 23% of the patients with both CP and MR and 10.9% of patients with MR had severe epilepsy. Table 2 shows the cases with CP and MR had a declining prevalence of epilepsy over the decades, compared to the controls. The test of trend demonstrates a statistically significant difference from trend of increasing prevalence in controls. It is noteworthy that the cases with autism and Down syndrome had a steadily increasing prevalence of epilepsy over the decades, and thus the test of trend was not statistically significantly different from controls.

Table 1. Prevalence of Epilepsy for patients without disability and developmental disability group, by known risk factors

All Cases of epilepsy	Without disability	All DD	Autism	Down Syndrome	Cerebral Palsy	MR with Psychiatric Illness	MR
	1809	694	54	58	163	152	267
All	1.0	27.0	24.1	13.8	36.8	22.4	27.0
Gender							
Male	1.0	24.9	28.6	8.8	39.2	21.6	22.1
Female	1.0	29.2	8.3	20.8	34.8	23.1	32.8
Race							
White	0.8	26.0	23.7	4.7	36.8	25.3	25.5
African American	1.2	28.3	20.0	42.9	35.7	19.5	30.0
Other	0.0	66.7	100.0	0.0	100.0	0.0	0.0
Severity of Primary Disability							
Mild	n/a	n/a	30.0	0.0	38.0	16.7	19.4
Moderate	n/a	n/a	23.1	12.5	35.7	33.3	26.7
Severe	n/a	n/a	20.0	15.9	36.8	29.3	33.9
Residential Type							
Least Restrictive Environment	n/a	23.2	0.0	16.7	35.0	30.4	18.5
Most Restrictive Environment	n/a	31.6	18.8	6.3	36.2	36.1	33.8

Table 2. Prevalence of all seizure severity combined, by developmental disability group, for each age group

All Seizures	20 - 29	30-40	40-50	50-60	60+
Comparison	0.97	0.79	1.28	1.42	0.00
Autism	27.50	0.00	20.00	50.00	0.00
Down Syndrome	7.14	7.69	33.33	25.00	0.00
Cerebral Palsy	35.37	47.37	39.28	20.00	0.00
MR with psychiatric Illness	23.64	26.32	19.35	17.65	18.18
MR Only	29.41	25.00	26.92	25.00	23.53

Table 3. Prevalence of severe seizures combined, by developmental disability group, for each age group

Severe Seizures Only	20 - 29	30-40	40-50	50-60	60+
Comparison	0.24	0.40	0.00	0.00	0.00
Autism	2.50	0.00	0.00	0.00	0.00
Down syndrome	0.00	0.00	0.00	0.00	0.00
Cerebral Palsy	8.54	7.89	3.57	0.00	0.00
MR with psychiatric Illness	0.00	0.00	0.00	0.00	0.00
MR Only	7.84	4.41	3.85	0.00	5.88

Figure 1 shows the prevalence in the controls and the case groups, from age 20 to 70+. The patients with CP and MR had the highest prevalence rates in three decades, 20-49 years. Patients with autism had the highest prevalence rates for the decade of 50-59 years and patients with Down syndrome had the highest prevalence in the decade 60-69 years.

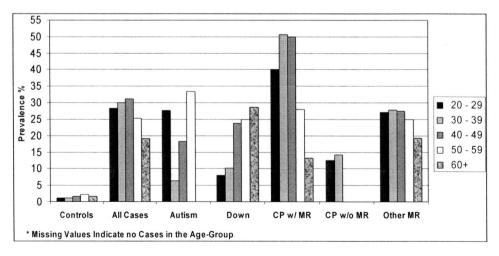

Figure 1. Prevalence of all seizure severity in patients without disabilities and by developmental disability group, by age group.

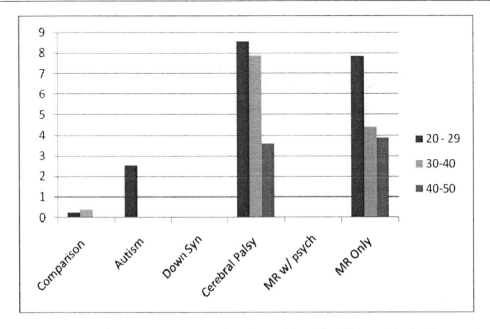

Figure 2. Prevalence of severe seizure severity in patients without disabilities and by developmental disability group, by age group.

Table 4 shows the odds ratio for epilepsy when we did not distinguish between moderate and severe cases. Only the group with cerebral palsy has statistically significantly higher risk compared to the patients without disability (Adjusted Odds Ratio 8.36 (95% Confidence Interval 1.03- 68.06) p=0.05).

When we explored the odds ratio for severe epilepsy the difference between those with autism, cerebral palsy and MR alone were statistically significantly higher compared to the group without disability. This is shown in Table 5. The adjusted odds ratio for adults with autism was 16.2, for those with cerebral palsy the odds ratio was 55.1 and for those with mental retardation the odds ratio was 41.4, compared to controls, after controlling for age, medical site, race, and gender.

Table 4. Logistic Regression, adjusted* odds ratio for prevalence of epilepsy by group

Groups	n	Prev.	Adjusted* Odds Ratio	Lower Confidence Interval	Upper Confidence Interval	P-Value
Comparison	1809	1.0	1.00			
Autism	54	24.1	3.95	0.43	36.37	0.225
Cerebral Palsy	**163**	**13.8**	**8.36**	**1.03**	**68.06**	**0.047**
Down syndrome	58	36.8	1.74	0.18	16.62	0.630
MR with Psychiatric Illness	152	22.4	4.15	0.47	36.44	0.198
MR Only	267	27.0	4.43	0.52	37.93	0.175

* adjusted for medical site, age, race, gender, tobacco use, and BMI.
Bold indicates statistically significantly different from comparison group.

Table 5. Logistic Regression, adjusted* odds ratio for prevalence of SEVERE epilepsy by group

Groups	n	Prev.	Adjusted* Odds Ratio	Lower Confidence Interval	Upper Confidence Interval	P-Value
Comparison	1809	0.17	1.00			
Autism	**54**	**1.85**	**16.16**	**1.44**	**181.17**	**0.024**
Cerebral Palsy	**163**	**6.75**	**55.09**	**11.78**	**257.60**	**0.001**
Down syndrome	58	0.00				
MR with Psychiatric Illness	152	0.00				
MR Only	**267**	**5.24**	**41.43**	**9.26**	**186.30**	**0.001**

* adjusted for medical site, age, race, gender.
Bold indicates statistically significantly different from the comparison group.

All patients with moderate and severe epilepsy were taking at least one antiepileptic medication. For moderate the top three medications were Carbamazepine, Phenytoin and Phenobarbital. For severe epilepsy the top three medications were Valproic Acid, Phenobarbital and Phenytoin (tied with Clonazepam). It should be noted that Vagal Nerve Stimulator was included as the only device in the list for severe epilepsy.

We used survival analysis to calculate incidence of epilepsy for those patients who entered the practices without established epilepsy. Hazard ratios for all the sub-groups are statistically significantly elevated, compared to the controls, ranging from a three fold higher rate of onset for adults with Down syndrome to 29 fold higher rate of onset for those with cerebral palsy compared to the comparison patients without disabilities (Table 6).

Table 6. Survival Analysis, adjusted* hazard rates for onset of epilepsy, among the developmental disability sub-groups compared to comparison patients

Groups	n	Hazard Ratio	P-Value
Comparison	1798		
Autism	**51**	**20.61**	**0.001**
Cerebral Palsy	**136**	**28.89**	**0.001**
Down syndrome	**56**	**3.69**	**0.001**
MR with Psychiatric Illness	**142**	**15.03**	**0.001**
MR Only	**236**	**19.24**	**0.001**

* adjusted for medical site, race, gender, tobacco use, BMI.
Bold indicates statistically significantly different from the comparison group.

Table 7 shows our calculated hazard ratios for the onset of severe epilepsy. The group with autism (Adjusted Hazard Ratio 12.4, p=0.02), cerebral palsy (Adjusted Hazard Ratio 52.2, p=0.001), and mental retardation (Adjusted Hazard Ratio 36.0, p=0.001) had substantially and statistically significantly higher rates of onset compared to the patients without disabilities.

Table 7. Survival Analysis, adjusted* hazard rates for onset of SEVERE epilepsy, among the developmental disability sub-groups compared to comparison patients.
(Severe cases of Epilepsy)

Groups	n	Hazard Ratio	P-Value
Comparison	1798		
Autism	**51**	**12.39**	**0.020**
Cerebral Palsy	**136**	**52.17**	**0.001**
Down syndrome	56		
MR with Psychiatric Illness	142		
MR Only	**236**	**36.01**	**0.001**

* adjusted for medical site, race, gender, tobacco use, BMI.
Bold indicates statistically significantly different from the comparison group.

Implications from our study findings: This study should provide some guidance to primary care physicians and other service providers about expected prevalence of epilepsy in adults with developmental disabilities, during six decades of life. Our study found an increasing prevalence of epilepsy, over the decades from age 20 to 60 years for the controls, and patients with Down syndrome and autism. It is noteworthy that those with MR and CP had a declining prevalence over the decades, similar to the results reported in the literature.

We compared the medication used by the patients in our study with a 1995 publication from the UK which used data from 119 general practitioners, and found the commonly used drugs were similar although there was variation in the proportion of patients on each drug (Hart and Shorvon et al, 1995). Since our study spanned decades we made the comparison to the 1995 since it represents a midpoint of our data. In our study more clonazepam, valproic acid, and phenobarital and less carbamazepine and phenytoin were used. The actual clinical management of our patient population is in keeping with the International Association for the Scientific Study of Intellectual Disabilities guidelines for the treatment of epilepsy. The guideline recommendations state that all individuals with seizures should be "assessed for accuracy of epilepsy diagnosis, appropriateness of current therapy and potential for improvement with further treatment" (IASSID et, 2002).

Implications for Case Study: The challenge of controlling LE's epilepsy have been substantial and a concerted effort was required from both the medical team and the staff who supported LE in her ICF/MR before her condition could be managed at an acceptable level. LE's severe epilepsy impacted her life and threatened her safety. It is important to help families and individuals with severe epilepsy establish a partnership with a physician in order to find a long term plan and to find a living situation where the individual can feel both comfortable and safe.

References

Acardi J. *Epilepsy in children.* 2nd Edition. New York: Raven Press; 1994.

Bowley C, Kerr M. Epilepsy and intellectual disability. *J. Intellect. Disabil. Res.,* 2000 44, 529-543.

Brodtkrob E. The diversity of epilepsy in adults with severe developmental disabilities: Age at seizure onset and other prognostic factors. *Seizure,* 1994 3, 277-285.

Deckers CL. Overtreatment in adults with epilepsy. *Epilepsy Res.* 2002 52, 43-52.

Devinsky O. What do you do when they grow up? Approaches to seizures in developmentally delayed adults. *Epilepsia* 2002 43, 71-79.

Deykin E, MacMahon B. The incidence of seizures among children with autistic symptoms. *Am. J. Psychiarty,* 1979 136, 1310-1312.

Hauser W. The prevalence and incidence of convulsive disorders in children. *Epilepsia,* 1994 35, S1-6.

IASSID. Health guidelines for adults with an intellectual disability, 2002. 2007 July 30. Available from: http://intellectualdisability.info/mental_phys_health/health_guide_adlt.htm.

Johannsen P, Christensen J. Epilepsy in Down syndrome-Prevalence in three groups. *Seizure,* 1996 5, 121-125.

Kotsoulos IA, van Merode T, Kessels FG, de Krom MC, Knottnerus JA. Systematic review of meta-analysis of incidence studies of epilepsy and unprovoked seizures. *Epilepsia,* 2002 43, 1402-1409.

McDermott S, Moran R, Platt T, Wood H, Isaac T, Dasari S. Prevalence of Epilepsy in adults with Mental Retardation and related disabilities in primary care. *Am. J. Ment. Retard.,* 2005 110, 48-56.

McVicker R, Shanks O, McClelland RJ. Prevalence and associated features of epilepsy in adults with Down syndrome. *B. J. Psychiatry,* 1994 164, 528-532.

Morgan C, Baxter H, Kerr M. Prevalence of epilepsy and associated health service utilization and mortality among patients with intellectual disability. *A. J. Ment. Retard.,* 2003 108, 293-300.

Mouridsen SE, Rich B, Isager T. Epilepsy in disintegrative psychosis and infantile autism: A long-term validation study. *Dev. Med. Child Neurol.,* 1999 41, 110-114.

National Institute of Health. May 13, 2007 Available from: http://www.ninds.nih.gov/disorders/epilepsy/epilepsy.htm

Pueschel SM, Louis S, McKnight P. Seizure disorders in Down syndrome. *Arch. Neurol,* 1991 48, 318–20.

Puri BK, Ho KW, Singh I. Age of seizure onset in adults with Down's syndrome. *Int. J. CLin. Pract.,* 2001 55, 442-444.

Singhi P, Jagirdar S, Khandelwal N, Malhi P. Epilepsy in children with cerebral palsy. *J. Child Nuerol.,* 2003 18, 174-179.

Tuchman R, Rapin I. Epilepsy in autism. *Lancet Nuerol.,* 2002 1, 352-58.

Volkmar F, Nelson DS. Seizure disorders in autism. *J. Am. Acad. Child Adolesc. Psychiatry,* 1990 29, 127-129.

World Health Organization. *International statistical classification of disease.* 9th edition. Geneva, Switzerland. 2000.

Chapter XIII

Death

The Research Questions: What is the age-specific death rate for adults with developmental disabilities and how do they differ from the comparison group?

Death Rates and Causes of Death in the General Population: The age-adjusted death rate for the United States, standardized to the year 2000 population, decreased from 832.7 deaths per 100,000 in 2003 to 801.0 deaths per 100,000 population in 2004. And the age-adjusted death rate declined significantly for 10 of the 15 leading causes of death. From 2003 to 2004, the preliminary age-adjusted death rate for the leading cause of death, diseases of heart, decreased by 6.4% and for cancer the decrease was 2.9%. Deaths from these two disease groupings combined accounted for more than 50% of all deaths in 2004 (Miniño, Heron, and Smith et al, 2006). Heart disease mortality has exhibited a downward trend since 1950 and cancer mortality has declined since 1990 (American Heart Association et al, 2002).

The leading causes of death have not changed in the past ten years although their ranking has varied. The 15 leading causes of death in 2004 were as follows: 1) Diseases of heart 2) Cancer 3) Cerebrovascular diseases 4) Chronic lower respiratory diseases (primarily Chronic Obstructive Pulmonary Disease) 5) Unintentional injuries 6) Diabetes mellitus 7) Alzheimer's disease 8) Influenza and pneumonia 9) Nephritis and other kidney disease 10) Septicemia;11) Intentional self-harm (suicide);12) Chronic liver disease and cirrhosis;13) Hypertension and hypertensive renal disease; 14) Parkinson's disease; and 15) Pneumonitis (Miniño, Heron, and Smith et al, 2006).

There are differences in mortality rates for different regions of the United States. Table 1 compares the mortality rate, by cause, for the US in general compared to South Carolina, where our study was conducted and the top six causes have the same rank.

Table 1. Age adjusted* mortality rate, by cause, for the US and South Carolina, 2003

Cause	US	South Carolina
All causes	832.7	934.8
Disease of the Heart	232.3	234.5
Cancer	190.1	203.3
Cerebrovascular Accident	53.5	69.0
Chronic Lower Respiratory	43.3	46.8
Diabetes Mellitus	25.3	28.0
Alzheimers	21.4	27.3

*Age Adjusted Rates per 100,000 population, 2003.

Literature Review of Death in Adults with Developmental Disability: The mortality rate of people with developmental disabilities is similar to the general population (Strauss and Eyman et al, 1996; Strauss and Kastner et al, 1996). And the experience of those with developmental disabilities is similar in that cardiovascular disease is the leading cause of death (Janicki, Dalton, and Henderson et al, 1999; Patja, Mölsä, and livanainen et al, 2001). The difference for those with DD is that there has not been a decrease in the proportion of overall deaths due to CVD; instead there has been a steady increase. Some recent reports suggest that CVD related deaths are greater for people with MR compared to the general population (Hill, Gridley, Cnattingius S et al. 2003; Day, Strauss, Shavelle, and Reynolds et al, 2005).

After adjusting for age, gender, and motor skills, adults with MR residing in community settings had a 72% higher overall mortality risk than adults with MR residing in an institution. In an Australian study, adults with MR have a higher mortality rate with significantly greater prevalence of no physical activity, obesity, and hypertension, compared to adults without MR (Beange, McElduff, and Baker et al, 1995; Strauss and Kastner et al, 1996; Strauss and Eyman et al, 1996).

To some degree the experience of people with developmental disabilities varies by impairment type. In the past decade and a half, investigators in a number of countries have noted a substantial improvement in the median age of death in individuals with Down syndrome (Leonard S, Bower, Petterson, and Leonard H et al, 2000) In a survey of 17,897 individuals with Down's syndrome compiled by the US Centers of Disease Control and Prevention National Center for Health Statistics for 1983–97, the median age of death increased from 25 years in 1983 to 49 years in 1997 (p<0·0001) When assessed by racial group, the median age of death was significantly higher in whites compared to African Americans and people of other races with Down syndrome. On the basis of data from death certificates, standardized mortality odds ratios (SMOR) of people with Down syndrome compared to those without DS, those with DS were more likely to show congenital heart defects SMOR (OR 29.1), dementia (OR 21.2), hypothyroidism (OR 20.3), or leukemia (OR 1.6). Apart from leukemia and testicular cancer, the SMORs for malignant diseases associated with Down syndrome were less than one-tenth as often as expected (0.07, 0.06-0.08) (Yang, Rasmussen, Friedman et al, 2002).

What is the Conceptual Framework for this question?: The life expectancy for people with developmental disabilities has dramatically improved in the past 30 years (Walz,1986; Patja, Molsa, Iivanainen, 2001). This is a related to more aggressive care for the newborn and young children with birth defects and the survival of people with acquired conditions, including injuries and medical conditions. In addition, individuals with developmental disability have a greater opportunity to participate in the community and family life and receive the community standard of medical care. The service system has developed a range of housing options, there are substantial improvements in both primary and specialty medical care, there are integrated employment options for adults with disabilities, and a variety of other options. It is well understood that some people with developmental disabilities associated with genetic syndromes have anomalies and medical conditions which require specialized care and in some cases the risk for premature mortality remains high. In other cases, people with developmental disabilities are protected from some of the risks faced by the age matched peers. People with DD are unlikely to be driving motor vehicles, they are constrained from some risky choices by caregivers and family, and they are often provided access to medical care through eligibility for Medicaid and to a lesser extent Medicare insurance. Thus, it is important to evaluate the question of whether age-adjusted mortality rates and causes of death are different for this group.

Case Study: JB is a 47 year old female with severe mental retardation (ICD9 318.1), Cerebral Palsy with hemiplegia (ICD9 343.1), and Grand Mal Seizure disorder (ICD9 345.10) treated with dilantin and valporic acid. In addition, she has the diagnosis of Gastroesophageal Reflux Disease (ICD9 530.81). Soon after family applied to the local disability service agency, when JB was 38 years of age, she was thoroughly evaluated and began seeing Dr. K., a family medicine physician at a University affiliated rural clinic. JB moved into a community based ICF-MR on the outskirts of the town where Dr. K. had his practice. He agreed to provide primary care and coordinate her specialist consultations. Initially after assuming responsibility for her care Dr. K. asked the staff to take notes to assess her eating, sleeping, and seizure patterns. From the notes it became clear that JB had some coughing when eating her meals. Dr. K. made a referral to a gastroenterologist for formal swallowing studies and it was determined that she was aspirating thin liquids. Her liquids were again thickened and delivered to her in a nectar consistency. In addition, JB was mute and communicated only by gesturing and groaning sounds. Despite this the staff felt they were able to anticipate and respond to her needs. JB was never hospitalized and rarely had any more than 2-3 seizures per year.

Dr. K. saw JB every two to three months when staff had concerns about breakdowns in her skin, suspicions about symptoms of colds, or other concerns. Dr. K. provided preventive services including influenza and pneumonia vaccination, screening for risk factors (e.g. cholesterol, blood pressure) and careful observation for changes in her health status.

Suddenly one day in May, JB was noted to be listless with a poor appetite at breakfast, but around mid-morning she suddenly collapsed at her ICF MR residence. She was minimally able to sit up and was not responsive at that time. The staff called the nursing staff who arrived at the house within 20 minutes. It was quickly determined that her temperature was 104 and she was transported by ambulance to the hospital. In the ER her evaluation indicated she had bilateral lower lobe pneumonia and a measurement of blood oxygen saturation (pulse oximetry reading) of 78% on room air. JB was immediately intubated and taken to the ICU where she remained minimally conscious. All efforts to treat her pneumonia failed and she died on hospital day 3, never regaining consciousness.

Our Research Findings: Death was recorded on the medical record when it occurred in the hospital when the individual was under the care of one of the physicians in the two practices, reported by a family member or staff member, or when it was identified in the National Death Index. We purchased the National Death Index from the National Center for Health Statistics at the end of the study to obtain information about death if it occurred for our case or comparison group. The study was reviewed by the NCHS Death Index review panel and the data were provided at the person level. The actual rates of occurrence of death are shown in Table 2 below.

The death rate for both the comparison group and our sub-groups with DD were extremely low since only 81 individuals in the comparison group and 20 individuals in all the DD groups died. Because of this we cannot reliably report on the causes of death, since despite use of the clinical record and the National Death Index the number of cases with an assigned cause of death less than 50 people.

We conducted survival analysis to determine if there were any differences in the rate of death between each of the developmental disability groups and the comparison group. First we also analyzed the risk factors for death in our dataset. As expected the risks for death were lower for women (Hazard Rate 0.49; p=0.001), higher for African-Americans compared to whites (Hazard Rate 1.61; p=0.04), higher for those with diabetes (Hazard Rate 1.69; p=0.026) and those who were smokers (Hazard Rate 1.72; p=0.017). None of the DD groups had statistically significantly higher death rates compared to the patients without disabilities, after controlling for these risk factors, as shown in Table 3.

Implications from our study findings: There were no statistically significant differences in the hazard ratio for death among the sub-groups of people with developmental disabilities compared to the comparison patients in the practice. This should allay some concerns among primary care practitioners about the type of care they need to provide to this special population. Patients in this study were on average approximately 40 years old when they entered care and with 7-10 years of follow-up death was a relatively rare event.

Implications for Case Study: The challenges for physicians and other providers of care and support for people with severe and profound developmental disabilities are complex. In fact most primary care physicians have very limited experience providing care for adults who are nonverbal and medically complex. Thus, as with many low incidence conditions a few physicians in any one community probably provide the majority of care to the people in this group. Changes in the individuals' condition can be subtle and therefore difficult to detect and without the subjective reports of change in pain or function even the most caring family and staff might not recognize an alternation. Death can be precipitous. A thorough medical post-mortem is important to determine if additional care or supports could have prevented the death.

Table 2. Death rates for people with no disability and developmental disabilities, by risk groups

prevalence (ever)	without disability	With DD	Autism	Down syndrome	Cerebral Palsy	MR w/ Psychiatric Illness	MR
All	1809	694	54	58	163	152	267
	4.5	2.9	1.9	3.6	1.8	3.3	3.4
Gender							
Male	5.8	3.8	2.4	5.9	2.7	2.7	4.8
Female	3.4	1.9	0.0	0.0	1.1	3.9	1.6
Race							
White	3.9	2.9	2.6	2.3	1.9	2.7	3.9
African American	5.3	2.9	0.0	7.1	1.8	3.9	2.7
Other	0	0.0	0.0	0.0	0.0	0.0	0.0
Severity of Primary Disability							
Mild	n/a	n/a	0.0	0.0	0.0	3.3	3.1
Moderate	n/a	n/a	2.6	12.5	1.8	4.8	5.0
Severe	n/a	n/a	0.0	2.3	3.5	2.4	2.8
Residential Type							
Least Restrictive Environment	n/a	1.8	0.0	0.0	0.0	4.4	1.9
Most Restrictive Environment	n/a	1.0	0.0	6.3	0.0	0.0	1.3

Table 3. Survival Analysis, Adjusted* Hazard Ratio for death, by sub-group with developmental disability compared to comparison patients

Groups	N	Hazard Ratio	P-Value
Comparison	1809		
Autism	54	2.03	0.488
Cerebral Palsy	163	0.56	0.421
Down syndrome	58	1.65	0.493
MR with Psychiatric Illness	152	0.53	0.216
MR Only	267	0.58	0.175

*adjusted for practice site, age, race, gender, and smoking.

References

American Heart Association. Heart disease and stroke statistics: 2003 update, 2002. 2007 July 30. Available from: http://www.americanheart.org/presenter.jhtml?identifier= 3007338.

Beange H, McElduff A, Baker W. Medical disorders of adults with mental retardation: a population study. *Am. J. Ment. Retard.,* 1995 99, 595-604.

Day SM, Strauss DJ, Shavelle RM, Reynolds RJ. Mortality and causes of death in persons with Down syndrome in California. *Dev. Med. Child Neurol.,* 2005 47, 171-176.

Hill DA, Gridley G. Mortality and cancer incidence among individuals with Down syndrome. *Arch. Intern. Med.,* 2003 163, 705-711.

Janicki MP, Dalton AJ, Henderson CM, Davidson PW. Mortality and morbidity among older adults with intellectual disability: health service considerations. *Disabil. Rehabil.,* 19991 21, 284-294.

Leonard S, Bower C, Petterson B, Leonard H. Survival of infants born with Down's syndrome. *Paediatr. Perinat. Epidemiol.,* 2000 14, 163-171.

Miniño AM, Heron MP, Smith BL. Deaths: preliminary data for 2004. 2007 July 30. Available from: http://www..cdc.gov/nchs/prodcuts/pubs/pubd/hestats/prelimdeath04/ preliminarydeaths2004.htm.

Patja K, Mölsä P, livanainen M. Cause-specific mortality of people with intellectual disability in a population-based, 25-year follow-up study. *J. of Intellectual Disability Research,* 2001, 45, 30-40.

Strauss D, Eyman RK. Mortality of people with mental retardation in California with and without Down syndrome. *Am. J. Ment. Retard.,* 1996 100, 643-653.

Strauss D, Kastner TA. Comparative mortality of people with mental retardation in institutions and the community. *Am. J. Ment. Retard.,* 1996 101, 26-40.

Walz T, Harper D, Wilson J. The aging developmentally disabled person a review. *Gerontologist,* 1986, 26, 622-629.

Yang Q, Rasmussen SA, Friedman JM. Mortality associated with Down's syndrome in the USA from 1983 to 1997: a population-based study. *Lancet,* 2002 359, 1019-1025.

Chapter XIV

Conclusion

This study was a thorough investigation into the primary care experience of a large group of adults with developmental disabilities from the vantage point of their medical home. The patients under observation were a mixture of individuals living in the community in a wide array of settings ranging from the least restrictive environments of independent living to the most restrictive environments of Intermediate Care Facilities for adults with mental retardation (ICF-MR). We also studied the longitudinal experience of a group of patients without disabilities who had the same medical homes. We believe this comparison minimized some of the subtle influences of practice patterns and community characteristics which might have influenced the results of previous studies.

It is clear that self-management of chronic conditions is highly influenced by living arrangements, social support, employment, income and education. People with developmental disabilities are at a clear disadvantage in all these domains. They are less likely to be living in a home of their choice, they have smaller circles of support, they are more likely to be unemployed and have low income, and clearly their intellectual disability is reflected in their low educational achievement. However, despite these disadvantages it is important to note that for most of the conditions we studied, people with developmental disabilities did not have higher prevalence compared to those without a disability (Tables 1 and 2).

Table 1. Conditions with *no statistically significant difference* in prevalence* for adults with developmental disabilities compared to adults with no disability

CONDITION	ODDS RATIO
Asthma	0.73 (0.47, 1.15) p=0.171
Congestive Heart Failure	1.15 (0.64, 2.09) p=0.644
Diabetes	1.14 (0.83, 1.57) p=0.408
Epilepsy	3.49 (0.40, 30.81) p=0.260
Hypertension	1.04 (0.27, 4.00) p=0.956
Obesity	0.86 (0.71, 1.04) p=0.125
Death	0.80 (0.45, 1.42) p=0.441

*Logistic regression adjusted odds ratio controlling for age, race, and gender.

Table 2. Conditions with *statistically significant lower* prevalence* for adults with developmental disabilities compared to adults with no disability

CONDITION	ODDS RATIO
Coronary Artery Disease	0.49 (0.26, 0.92) p=0.027
Depression	0.73 (0.57, 0.92) p=0.009

*Logistic regression adjusted odds ratio controlling for age, race, and gender.

Table 1 shows the conditions where there was no statistical difference between the prevalence of the common health conditions for the group with developmental disabilities and the comparison patients.

Table 2 shows the conditions where the patients with developmental disabilities had lower prevalence of the common health conditions compared to the comparison patients.

Epilepsy was an interesting condition since the prevalence was not significantly different when all severity levels of epilepsy were considered. However, when we looked at severe epilepsy, which was defined as epilepsy that was challenging to control with at least two medications, there was higher prevalence among the group with developmental disabilities. In addition to severe epilepsy there were two other conditions, dementia and chronic obstructive pulmonary disease, for which individuals with developmental disabilities had higher prevalence than individuals without DD. The results are shown in Table 3.

Many people come to family medicine practices with previously diagnosed conditions thus we also explored the onset of each of the conditions among the patients who entered the practices without an established diagnosis. Again, the risk of developing the conditions was more likely to be no different for those with developmental disabilities compared to those without disabilities (Table 4).

Table 5 shows that the risk for onset of Coronary Artery Disease was statistically significantly lower for people with developmental disabilities compared to those without a disability. This hazard ratio is substantially lower and it conveys a clinically significant reduction in risk.

For those who entered the practices without a condition only dementia and epilepsy had higher onset for adults with developmental disabilities compared to those without disability (Table 6).

Table 3. Conditions with *statistically significant higher* prevalence* for adults with developmental disabilities compared to adults with no disability

CONDITION	ODDS RATIO
Chronic Obstructive Pulmonary Disease	1.71 (1.19, 2.58) p=0.011
Dementia	9.95 (5.38, 18.40) p=0.001
Severe Epilepsy	21.98 (4.94, 97.72) p=0.001

* Logistic regression adjusted odds ratio controlling for age, race, and gender.

Table 4. Conditions with *no statistically significant difference* in onset* for adults with developmental disabilities compared to adults with no disability

CONDITION	HAZARD RATIO
Asthma	0.80 p=0.305
Congestive Heart Failure	0.82 p=0.477
Chronic Obstructive Pulmonary Disease	1.04 p=0.816
Depression	0.82 p=0.076
Diabetes	0.96 p=0.782
Hypertension	0.88 p=0.151
Obesity	1.07 p=0.195
Death	0.86 p=0.121

* Survival analysis controlling for age, race and gender.

Table 5. Condition with *statistically significant lower* onset* for adults with developmental disabilities compared to adults with no disability

CONDITION	HAZARD RATIO
Coronary Artery Disease	0.36 p=0.001

* Survival analysis controlling for age, race and gender.

Table 6. Conditions with *statistically significant higher* onset* for adults with developmental disabilities compared to adults with no disability

CONDITION	HAZARD RATIO
Dementia	6.07 p=0.001
Epilepsy	28.43 p=0.001
Severe Epilepsy	31.99 p=0.001

* Survival analysis controlling for age, race and gender.

Another way to look at the results of our study is to see what was statistically significantly different for each of the case groups compared to the comparison group. The details of these findings are in the preceding chapters. The summary of those results are described as risk for onset among those entering care without the conditions (Survival Analysis results described with the Hazard ratio) and the risk for ever having the condition (Logistic Regression results described with the Odds ratio):

- Autism: higher risk for onset of obesity and epilepsy and severe epilepsy, lower risk for prevalence of COPD among people who never smoked, and higher risk for prevalence of severe epilepsy.
- Down syndrome: higher risk for onset of obesity, dementia, and epilepsy; higher risk for prevalence of obesity and dementia.
- Cerebral palsy: higher risk for onset of epilepsy and severe epilepsy; higher risk for prevalence of dementia, epilepsy and severe epilepsy; lower risk for onset of obesity

and depression; lower risk for prevalence of depression, obesity, and COPD among those who never smoked.

- Mental retardation with psychiatric illness: higher risk for onset of dementia and epilepsy; higher risk for prevalence of dementia, and lower risk for onset of CAD.
- Mental retardation: higher risk for onset of dementia, epilepsy and severe epilepsy; higher risk for prevalence of dementia, COPD and epilepsy; lower risk for onset of CAD and COPD for those who never smoked; lower risk for prevalence of depression.

The limitations of this study include concern about sample size and the power to find a difference in odds for occurrence of each of the health conditions for those with autism, cerebral palsy and Down syndrome compared to our comparison group. We were limited by the number of individuals at our sites with these conditions but we hope other research groups will repeat this study with more study participants. In addition, the retrospective record review only allowed us to only use information that was systematically collected in the clinical setting, so we did not have data about many other parameters that could impact the results. These parameters include some diagnostic test results, measures of health promoting behaviors such as physical activity and diet, measures of social, emotional, behavioral, and knowledge domains, and presence or absence of a number of other health conditions and risk factors. A prospective study is needed to capture a larger array of factors. Finally, we limited our study to two primary care sites and the results could be geographically specific. Repeating the study at other sites is needed before the results can be generalized.

For researchers interested in understanding the specific differences between adults with DD and their same age peers there remain a large number of unanswered questions. For example: (1) are there some other conditions that are substantially more prevalent in people with DD? (2) are there other conditions, like dementia for adults with Down syndrome, where the onset is substantially different? (3) are there different responses to treatments for the groups ?, (4) are there approaches to care that are more effective for any of the cases groups compared to the comparison patients? Some of these questions can be answered using comparable datasets to the one we used. Other questions will need a randomized intervention trial format to find the answer.

Only dementia and severe epilepsy have both statistically significantly higher odds ratios for prevalence and larger hazard ratios for onset, among adults with developmental disabilities during the seven to ten years of primary care follow-up. Chronic Obstructive Pulmonary Disease had a higher odds ratio, but no difference in the onset among the adults with developmental disabilities compared to adults without disabilities.

The most compelling finding of our study is that when comparisons are made to people in the same socioeconomic environment there are only a few conditions that disproportionately impact people with developmental disabilities, when we can control for some of the established risk factors. In addition, we found that individuals with developmental disabilities who were obese when they entered care at the two medical sites were more likely to return to normal weight compared to the comparison patients. This is an optimistic finding for doctors, patients and care providers.

This study compared adults living in the same communities and in the same medical practices which reduces the bias in environmental exposures and practice patterns. When this is done the differences between adults with developmental disabilities and their same age peers are negated. In fact coronary artery disease had lower prevalence and incidence for the adults with developmental disabilities and depression had lower prevalence for the DD group. For the chronic conditions of asthma, congestive heart failure, diabetes, hypertension, obesity and even death there was no difference in prevalence or onset between the DD and the comparison groups.

Appendix A
Residential Options for Adults

Community Training Home I (CTH I)

1. Caregivers are contracted by the Provider
2. Services are provided in the caregiver's home
3. Limited to a maximum 2-bed capacity for consumers. Exceptions may be made for increased bed capacity (not to exceed 3-beds for consumers) if the caregiver has worked with two consumers for six months.
4. Services and supports required by consumers vary in degree from consumer to consumer.
5. Consumers receive habilitation services to increase independent living skills and/or to prevent regression
6. When consumers are present, a qualified caregiver is required to be on-site to supervise and provide services.
7. Qualified caregivers are available 24 hours, seven days a week, 365-days a year, to provide supports
8. Manufactured or mobile homes may be used when serving 2 or less consumers.
9. The home shall not admit individuals placed in the home by other agencies, unless prior approval is granted by SCDDSN.
10. Complies with SCDDSN Residential Habilitation Standards
11. Certified every three years by SCDDSN

Community Training Home II (CTH II)

1. Caregivers are employed by the Provider
2. Services are provided in a home that is owned or managed by the Provider.
3. Limited to a maximum 4-bed capacity for consumers
4. Services and supports required by consumers vary in degree from consumer to consumer.

5. Consumers receive habilitation services to increase independent living skills and/or to prevent regression
6. When a consumer is present in the home, a qualified caregiver is required to be in the home and awake to supervise and provide services.
7. Qualified caregivers are available 24 hours, seven days a week, 365-days a year, to provide supports
8. Manufactured homes or trailers cannot be used unless the State Fire Marshal approves an alternative method of compliance.
9. A type "13" sprinkler system must be installed when serving 4 consumers not independent in self-preservation within 3 minutes of a fire-drill, unless the State Fire Marshal approves an alternative method of compliance.
10. The home shall not admit individuals placed in the home by other agencies, unless prior approval is granted by SCDDSN.
11. Complies with SCDDSN Residential Habilitation Standards
12. Certified every three years by SCDDSN

Supervised Living Program I (SLP I)

1. Any home, apartment or condominium owned or leased by the consumer.
2. Manufactured or mobile homes may be used when serving 2 or less consumers.
3. Limited to a 2-bed maximum capacity for consumers.
4. Consumers are at least 18 years of age; able to complete most of their activities of daily living skills with periodic supports from caregivers; able to evacuate independently, and have sufficient financial resources to meet basic expenditures.
5. Consumers receive habilitation services to increase independent living skills and/or to prevent regression.
6. Qualified caregivers are available 24 hours, seven days a week, 365-days a year, to provide supports, but are not required to be stationed on-site.
7. The home shall not admit individuals placed in the home by other agencies, unless prior approval is granted by SCDDSN.
8. Complies with SCDDSN Residential Habilitation Standards.
9. Inspected every three years by SCDDSN.

Supervised Living Program II (SLP II)

1. Any home, apartment or condominium owned or leased by the consumer.
2. Manufactured homes or trailers cannot be used unless the State Fire Marshal approves an alternative method of compliance.
3. Limited to a 3-bed maximum capacity for consumers.
4. Consumers are able to complete some of their activities of daily living skills with intermittent supports from caregivers; at least 18 years of age; able to evacuate independently, and have sufficient financial resources to meet basic expenditures.

5. Consumers receive habilitation services to increase independent living skills and/or to prevent regression.
6. When consumers are present, qualified caregivers are required to be awake and on-site.
7. Qualified caregivers are available 24 hours, seven days a week, 365-days a year, to provide supports.
8. The home shall not admit individuals placed in the home by other agencies, unless prior approval is granted by SCDDSN.
9. Complies with SCDDSN Residential Habilitation Standards.
10. Inspected every three years by SCDDSN.

Waiver Respite Home or Facility

1. Provided in most residential or day facilities owned by the consumer, caregiver or Provider.
2. Caregivers can be selected by the consumer or the Provider.
3. Services are provided to consumers who are unable to care for themselves, because of the absence or need for relief of those persons normally providing the care and supervision.
4. Used only for short term, temporary care.
5. Services and supports required by consumers vary in degree from consumer to consumer.
6. Licensed respite homes are limited to a maximum 2-bed capacity for consumers. For all other licensed or certified residential or day facilities, only the maximum number of consumers identified on the certificate and/or license can be served.
7. When consumers are present, qualified caregivers are available to provide supervision and services.
8. Complies with SCDDSN Respite Standards.
9. Inspected annually by the Provider every two consecutive years, and licensed by SCDDSN every third year.

Index

B

C

D

T

U

V

W

Y